The Opioid Labyrinth: A Search for Solutions Beyond the Statistics

Nancy

Table of Contents

Preface. Adam

As he eased into his chair, I could immediately tell he was exhausted. Adam had just recently started a job working third shift at a shipping warehouse and was still getting accustomed to working nights. Living in a halfway house didn't make things any easier. The small bunkroom where he was housed was loud, a constant bustling in the background punctuated by the sounds of whatever movie was playing on the television. Everyone in the treatment program was housed here, a space no bigger than the average waiting room packed with prison-style bunks from wall to wall. Having upwards of 20 men in a space this small made catching up on sleep during the day an aspirational task, but it didn't keep them from trying. Many had towels draped over the edges of the top bunk to try to at least block out the fluorescent lights that never turned off.

When they weren't going to treatment or work, this is where they stayed. No one was allowed to leave. The administrators of the facility tried as hard as they could to keep them secluded, away from the hundreds of other men they housed in other wings residing there for offenses that didn't land them in treatment. In this facility, it was common knowledge that you could get just about any drug you wanted. "It's why they never let us leave," he says. While Adam had been clean for four months and his Vivitrol shot helped to cancel out most of what remained of his cravings, for those in the earlier stages of the program, sobriety was a new experience. Just knowing that you could get exactly what you wanted *just* like that meant they had to isolate you. The temptation was too strong.

It was like that in the early stages for Adam. He'd been staying here for about three months, long enough to acclimate and get to the point where he considered several of his classmates to be real friends. Having spoken to so many of them, this was rare. Most of the guys preferred to keep each other at arm's length, regarding others mostly as acquaintances. That wasn't Adam. Even on only a few hours' sleep, beanie nearly pulled down over his eyes, his affability came through. It was no surprise that, in what seemed like a past life, Adam had always made friends easily. He'd spent years doing stand-up comedy after a broken foot derailed a burgeoning professional skating career that began in his adolescent years. Losing skating was a blow. As a teenager, he travelled constantly, relishing the opportunity to stay on the move for most of the year. Even though he was frequently on the road, he was a good student and maintained his grades. During high school, almost all of his friends smoked weed and drank, but none of that appealed to him. While he admits he'd occasionally get into trouble, it was from his hyper nature, not for drinking or drugs. Unlike so many teenagers, he even had a mind to wait to have his first drink until he was 21 despite having ample opportunity.

Adam spent the next handful of years traveling doing stand-up off and on, picking up odd jobs here and there to make ends meet along the way. For most of the year he lived by himself in a nice neighborhood slightly removed from the city that had an eclectic, blue-state vibe in the middle of a red state. Overall, Adam was doing well. Money wasn't a problem, and his bills were always paid. He eventually settled into a job as a chef at a local bar and enjoyed it, staying longer than he had with other jobs in the past. True to his character, he hung out with a lot of different sorts of crowds in his time off, "Musicians, punk rocker people or different musician people. Artsy people. Just weird people, skating people, my comedy friends, just friends from school that I've kept in touch with. Random people…All different genres of people."

Around 2009, he began to notice that pills were starting pop up more frequently. The weird part, he thought, was that it wasn't isolated just to one or two social circles– they were everywhere. "I slowly started to see that opioids trickled into every one of those groups…no matter who they were or what backgrounds were." Adam knew that they were percs (Percocet) right away. He'd intermittently had prescriptions for them since he broke his foot years ago to help cope with residual pain. He never had a problem with them up to that point, only using them as intended. But as they became increasingly popular and flooded the local market, like his friends, he started taking them more frequently.

It started slowly, taking one, maybe two in a day. Only eating them. But then one or two became three or four, which became five or six. A friend told him that if you crush them up and snort them it was even better. They were right. Snort one, eat one. Do that a few times a day. This continued for several months, escalating in small, imperceptible steps. Eventually, he paused, thinking back on how he'd gotten to where he was, "About eight to 10 months in…I started doing 15 pills per day and I remembered when half of one pill used to make me puke and I'd nod out on just one. And then sniffing 15 of them or shooting seven of them at a time and nothing going on. Just a little mild buzz and then just not sick for a few hours." Your body quickly builds a tolerance to opioids and this was becoming evident for Adam. What began as an inexpensive, potent habit had become something that his body barely registered. Soon, he found himself chasing that same feeling he had when his use started,

> "That's why I increased taking more and more of them. I just knew I was building up a tolerance. Once that warm feeling goes away, that high feeling…it wasn't a maintenance thing at that point yet. It was just, I'll just do it because it's there and since I can afford it, since I've got hundreds of them, why not do as many until I feel it? That should do something. But then when it doesn't, because I wasn't taking 15 a day for very long before it was, this is $300, $400 a day."

Adam had been getting his pills from a variety of sources. His most reliable, a 60-year-old man he knew that was getting 120 a month for some reason or another. He'd give him $1,000 and they were his– worth considerably more on the street. At one point, they'd reach $1/mg and 120 perc 30s meant there was a lot of money in that small orange bottle. He was getting his own script too. He'd do some, sell some. It was a fluid process where there were always pills and there was always cash. Finding a market for them was easy with as many friends as he had. Demand was high and getting them at a steep discount or from his pharmacy subsidized his dealings.

As his tolerance continued to increase, there was a point where the percs just didn't seem worth it. Why spend all of this money on something that barely does anything? The cost/benefit just wasn't there anymore, so he decided it was time to stop. That way, he thought, he'd have even more pills he could sell. But quitting percs cold turkey turned out to be a significantly different experience than he anticipated, "I didn't realize I had become addicted until I decided to stop taking them one day…I told my friend I felt like shit. He's, 'Oh, well you're dope sick.' I said, 'Well, I don't even do heroin,' and he said, 'Well, you get it from them pills too.'" It was at this point that Adam realized that he "might have fucked up." Taking them until he'd feel something had deepened his body's need for them. He'd never been sick before. In the year or so that he'd been doing them, supply was never a problem, "they were always there. It wasn't really an issue. I never even thought about it…it really never crossed my mind."

When he started taking the percs recreationally, he didn't think twice. In his eyes, they weren't *really* drugs. After all, they came from a pharmacy. A doctor wouldn't write someone a script with seemingly endless refills if it was addictive or bad for you, right?

Why would they give you something like this and keep prescribing it to somebody? Because I was selling them from 2011. I was getting them from the same guy who was getting them from his doctor from 2011 to 2015. One hundred and twenty of them. I thought if they're going to prescribe him these then why would you give them to somebody for so long if that's not necessary, especially in that large amount? I thought, 'Oh, they're from a doctor so they'll be fine.' And I really thought you could only get dope sick from doing heroin…I didn't think it would be how it was.

Many have asked similar questions in recent years, trying to determine how much prescribers are to blame for the flood of opioid painkillers and the damage they've created, but for Adam, the who or why weren't important. All he knew was that he was dope sick– sweating, shaking, vomiting, diarrhea– and it was a problem. The pills were getting too expensive, and the more he required for himself, the less money he made selling. On top of not feeling much from them anymore, he was getting sick faster and was starting to get uneasy about his situation for the first time. Noticing changes in him, some of Adam's friends, also opioid users, started to nudge him towards an alternative. There was something else that was just as easy to get, was cheaper, and lasted longer.

Adam graduated to heroin a little over a year into his opioid use. The decision was simple and required little deliberation, "I pretty much switched to heroin because the pills were, for me to do $180 worth of pills just to feel good for four hours, where I could do $20 worth of heroin and be good for 18 and 20 hours." At first, heroin wasn't about getting high. It was about staying well. He'd be able to avoid the crippling sickness for the entire day and have extra cash from selling more pills– win-win.

When Adam was on percs, he lived comfortably. The income he received from selling, on top of what he made at his job, left him able to do just about anything he wanted. Things got a bit tighter towards the end, hence the switch to heroin, but it never got to where he was really ever desperate. Similar to his trajectory with percs, Adam started using more heroin, bit by bit. The first few months were uneventful, but there reached a point where things began to deteriorate rapidly. He was burning through his savings and selling the assets he'd accumulated in a way that he hadn't had to before, "I didn't really start selling stuff until I was doing heroin. I had plenty of money when I was doing Percocet. That was never an issue."

Around the time he started using heroin, to no fault of his own, his world began to crumble even further. He learned that the restaurant where he managed the kitchen was going out of business, leaving him unemployed. It didn't faze him much at first, thinking he'd get another job quickly. He didn't. Instead, more went wrong. On Father's Day, he learned that his dad had terminal cancer. He'd die only 16 days later.

The news of his dad's diagnosis hit Adam like a ton of bricks, but his death so soon thereafter destroyed him. He was incredibly close with him and facing the reality that he'd passed was beyond what he could handle, "that's when I started doing four or five grams of heroin a day…everything just kind of spiraled out of control at the same time. And I just really didn't care." The heroin made his feelings go away, and, at that time, that was the ultimate draw. It was injectable indifference. Four to five grams of heroin is a *lot* of heroin, and it only accelerated his decline.

Only a few months after quitting the percs, he was right back to where he had started, spending a small fortune on opioids each day. What had initially begun as the budget-conscious option had become a considerable expense and not buying was not an option. Once again, he found himself battling increasingly frequent withdrawal symptoms, but this was a different kind of dope sick, a much worse kind of dope sick. Now, he was needle sick. He'd already been shooting pills, so he wasn't scared of the needle like he once was. But shooting heroin had pushed his dependence into uncharted territory and brought new levels of desperation with it, "It escalated pretty quickly. You're just selling things to get whatever the next fix is so you're not sick. You're basically- selling my guns, computers, whatever. Anything. Quit paying the bills or paying the bills late or not paying the full amount. Because the first like five years I lived there by myself everything was paid. I had no issues."

Adam knew what was happening. He saw it all, dating back to the first time he got sick off the percs. Unlike most addicts, he maintained an uncommon awareness to the realities of his ever-devolving situation. He continuously juxtaposed what had been only a year prior to where he was now,

> It was total clarity. I wasn't lying to myself. I knew I was a drug addict, and I knew what it was affecting. I knew what it was costing me. I was totally aware the whole time. There was no point where I was disillusioned...Honestly, the first couple of weeks after I realized I was getting sick from not taking the pills– that's what it was and really how severe it was. The first couple of times I tried to quit, that's when I was, "Well, it's pretty much game over." I knew the repercussions and what was happening because it was right in front of me. You had to be blind not to see it or just totally oblivious to the situation, which I don't see how you can. If you hadn't had a normal life before, you wouldn't know what you're missing out on. I knew from the beginning.

His sense of clarity was a double-edged sword. He understood the path he was on and where it led, but he was also able to recognize that quitting would be a herculean task. He knew that breaking his opioid dependence might not be in the cards– it might be too powerful, too daunting. Though, getting clean meant the chance to regain who he used to be and that was incentive enough to try.

Adam's desire to quit was sincere, but it was more complicated than that. He had always struggled with mental illness. In the past, he'd been content with his life, but depression had a propensity to creep in during those times when things grew stagnant or he wasn't staying busy.

That made heroin his worst enemy. The drugs changed him. His disgust of having moved to heroin, and the need to keep doing it, made him isolate. He withdrew from others as he slipped deeper into depression. He wasn't the same outgoing, gregarious person that he used to be. Even on the pills, he was able to maintain the part of him that thrived off an active social life, but he was different now, "I was always out in the mix, the life of the party, doing stuff like that and then to be a hermit and a reclusive was probably the thing that hurt me the most because I like to be around people."

His dad's death still dogged him and sitting at home in an empty apartment high on heroin wasn't helping matters. He was having trouble shaking the fact that he had to shoot up before the funeral just to be well enough to attend. Dwelling on the extent that opioids had permeated his life slowly chipped away at what was left of his mental health. Every once in a while, he'd hit a breaking point and decide he'd give quitting another go. Similar to many times before, the plan was to slowly taper himself down. To start smoking it instead of shooting it so the withdrawals wouldn't be as intense. Adam always struggled making it over that first hurdle, "after three, maybe four days, usually never got to four days. I would just give in because it definitely gets worse before it gets better." The small failures made a bad situation worse as they accumulated. Each one was another affirmation of how hard it was going to be to ever get out from under his addiction, the stress of which, paradoxically, made him use more, "I would try to use less and then I would not be successful so I would use more and that's where it would just go around, around, around."

Adam wasn't alone in his heroin use. The downside of being an outgoing person with a large friend network of 30-somethings in Ohio around 2014 was that your Facebook feed was constantly filled with news of someone you knew overdosing and dying. Stuck in a downward spiral, and already fragile, every bit of bad news was another trigger, "I had a bunch of friends dying at that time too from ODing that were people I've known for my whole life. So, it just became a vicious circle of the same shit every day, trying to deal with it. And then it seems when I get to a point where everything would be okay, I'm going to really try to quit again, something else would happen."

The cumulative effects of his cyclical failures exacerbated his already growing sense of apathy. Things mattered a lot less. Along the way, the threat of getting locked up didn't have the same effect that it used to. He just didn't care anymore. Heroin isn't cheap when you're using as much as he was, and Adam needed money. His new plan was to buy fake money off of Amazon and use it to buy gift cards to trade for dope. The crazy thing is it worked. At least that's what he thought at the time,

> Three weeks later the secret service came to my house. And that's when I got that
> F5 for forgery. And then I got an F5 for possession four months later. And I
> hadn't been in trouble in 14 years. And at that point I was, 'Now that I have a
> felony, this is affecting my life negatively for something that's very serious. So
> now it's time to start thinking about really quitting.' And that's when I asked my
> probation officer if I could go to rehab and I said, 'I can't quit on my own.'

An F5 (Felony 5) is the least severe category of felony in Ohio, nevertheless, a felony is a felony. Even though he didn't care about getting caught at first, these arrests mark when the severity of his situation really began to sink in. He'd had a few short stays in jail, but nothing like this. These charges could potentially land him in prison for several years, serving as a bit of a wake-up call. In the end, he was in jail again and this was a good thing.

> If I wouldn't have gone to jail, I probably wouldn't have quit because I always
> somehow would have the means to do it [use heroin] and I wanted to go to jail

and get into a program because I knew that would be the only way I quit. Because I knew once I could get over that first even week or 10 days, I knew I would never want to pick it up again…I was in jail before this last time. All I thought about is "I'm going to go get high as soon as I get out of here," but this last time…too much shit has happened. I'm almost 40. I got nothing going on anymore. I hang out with the same five fucking people. It's ridiculous. I would rather have just died and been happier.

Being incarcerated gave him time to get clean, clear his head, and not just think about his past, but to also start to see what could be in his future.

Adam could never get over that early-withdrawal hump. With the freedom to go get dope, it was too easy to be able to press a button and instantly make everything feel alright again. That option wasn't on the table anymore and he knew that's what he needed. Getting arrested and going through withdrawal wasn't a silver bullet, but it gave him a chance. It was an opportunity he just wasn't ready for the other times he'd been locked up. He had wanted to keep using, so he kept using. For all intents and purposes, having already given up on life made an arrest no longer have meaning. What was he afraid of losing? Getting out and getting well was the only thing on his mind. But this time, he knew things were different.

Many opioid addicts say that they've hit what they consider to be rock bottom. It's an imprecise term. Addicts will often have many bottoms. It's hard to distinguish which low was truly the worst of them all, or as one participant aptly put it, they're "just different shades of shit." While pinpointing his true bottom is difficult, Adam had hit what would turn out to be his last bottom. He was done.

Adam was determined to make a change. He'd asked his PO for help and he was going to get it. It was a long-term, three-month inpatient program that would teach him coping skills and cognitive behavioral techniques focused on identifying the triggers of his use. To someone that wanted help for several years, having a spot in the program was seen as a privilege. Throughout the program, he worked to fortify the barrier in his mind that separated then from now. Now, he was ready for what was next, "I was tired, I was sick of doing it. It was just exhausting…I was happy. It sucked to be in jail, but at least I know that this is the end. It's *done*. I can start really getting my life back and taking the steps to get back to where I was. I was definitely glad it happened. It sucked at the time, but looking back now, it's totally what I wanted." Adam finished his treatment program over the next six weeks and was released. Having finally gotten the help that he'd long wanted, he was eager to have a chance at a fresh start. Three days later, Adam was dead.

One of Many

Adam's story isn't special. He's just one of countless people in Ohio who have succumbed to opioid addiction. Members of the treatment community often say that 9 out of 10 addicts currently in treatment will relapse, often within the first year (Smyth et al. 2010). There's little reason to expect another outcome. On average, participants in my sample had just under *seven* separate periods of opioid addiction, consuming, at times, decades of individuals' lives as they struggled with the cycle of addiction. Use, get clean, relapse, and repeat until it either kills you or you reach a point where the personal and collateral damage reaches a critical mass that leads to lasting sobriety. Even then, maintaining that success is fleeting and often doesn't correlate with a lack of desire.

None of the guys still in Adam's program could say for certain what killed him. They could only speculate. The running suspicion was it was fentanyl. Maybe he knew what it was, maybe he didn't. It's become infamous for a reason- it's incredibly potent, up to 50 times stronger than heroin, but also volatile. More so than heroin, it's hard to gauge its strength. Unbeknownst to a user, it may also be mixed into something else, making shooting anything these days a modified game of Russian roulette.

What many didn't know at the time, was that Adam had been in contact with one of his drug connections the last few days he was still in the halfway house. Only six weeks prior, he spoke with such conviction that he was done. In spite of the strength of his commitment, as he neared release, he knew what he was going to do as soon as he set foot outside the facility. He'd changed his mind. He wasn't done.

In the brief moment between learning that someone in the program had died and finding out it was Adam, my mind jumped to who might have been the most likely candidate. As morbid of an exercise as it was, there were many in the class considerably younger than Adam and significantly less mature. Most didn't have the same kind of foresight he had; the kind that could recognize that continuing his addiction would lead nowhere good. Adam told me about several people that he thought didn't want to be in the program. They didn't really want help, at least not yet. They were there because it meant sidestepping a felony or a prison number. It bothered him. He didn't want people there that weren't on the same page as he was, and even talked about how they could be weeded out in the future. It would be hard, but he thought he had the answer, "If you just sit down and listen to somebody's story, you can tell if they're being genuine or not. So, for me, that's probably the only way that you can tell is how honest they are…Because if you're going to make up that big of a story to lie and convince somebody that you do want help and you really don't, then you're a *psychopath*."

So, was Adam a psychopath? No. At least I don't think so. Maybe I have to think that. I thought he was genuine and then he was gone. More than anything, Adam's story is a testament to the power of opioids, and heroin in particular. A person can have complete certainty that they're done. They can back it up with months of dedicated work to treat their addiction, but once an addict's brain expects the next dose, it will never be the same. Logic and reason have little, if any, role to play anymore. Using becomes a compulsion, amplifying the voice of the devil on their shoulder until it's the only thing they can hear. The cycle can be broken, but a person has to want it and they will likely need help to do it, but even then, as in Adam's case, it might not be enough. Ultimately, as Adam said, "You don't know what's going on in their head."

Like Any Other Person

The individuals that I had the privilege of interviewing came from all walks of life. Some were former million-dollar business owners, stay-at-home moms, career drug dealers, Marine Corps veterans, or blue-collar workers. They came from upper-class suburbs and the most rundown neighborhoods in Columbus. Some had records, some didn't. It didn't matter. Opioids took them all down the same. For my participants, stopping at recreational use was untenable, and their habits often escalated to the upper limits of tolerable toxicity. In that sense, it bears noting the difference between my sample and the millions of Americans who still have half-a-bottle of percs tucked away in a medicine cabinet with a dispose-by date long since passed. Given the disparity in the number of "as-directed" users and those that developed advanced addictions, it's easy to draw a line between yourself and "them," to dehumanize them. To say, "They're weak-willed and they should just quit." I've heard it. Honestly, I've thought it. But it's more complicated than that. We don't like complicated. Rather than dismissing their experiences as a matter of insufficient fortitude, there is much to be gained from an examination of how the worst-off users arrived at that destination. Marginalizing addicts obscures the events that have transpired in their lives that help to explain how their trajectories unfolded, factors that are essential to effectively addressing the opioid epidemic. The truth is that many of the individuals featured here are more like you than you'd care to think, and that's an unsettling notion– that if your life had played out slightly differently, that this could have been your story.

The Daily Cycle of Addiction

The consequences and innumerable indignities that accompany advanced opioid addiction can only be described as hell on earth. No one should dismiss the reality that there's a reason why people continue to use opioids in the early stages predating full-fledged addiction. Opioids produce a kind of high that many drugs can't match, but what often begins as wanting to have a good time or feel better about a trying time can devolve into the deepest, darkest point in a person's life where the phrase "I just want to die" is commonplace. By this stage, using isn't pleasurable. At least not like it used to be. Making sure you stay well is a job. Having become physically dependent, your body needs opioids to function properly. Go without, and you risk the onset of physical symptoms that render you incapable of the simplest tasks.

The life of an opioid addict becomes simple– get high, do anything necessary to find more, then do it again. As soon as the drugs are gone, the clock starts ticking. Focus shifts, knowing that withdrawal is lurking somewhere in the not-so-distant future. Depending on the strength of their last dose, it could be an hour, maybe three or four. Maybe more if they were especially lucky. But for seasoned users, that would be wishful thinking. The magnitude of the necessity of avoiding the sickness is difficult to comprehend. Most users have a hard time articulating the gravity of impending withdrawal symptoms, but the signs were readily apparent: the ominous change in tone, the uneasy shifts in posture, the change in their faces– half wry smile, half complete dread. Time and again I'd be asked if I had ever used. I'd shake my head and they would tell me how I'd never be able to understand.

> Have you ever been dope sick before? You'll never get it if you don't go through it. It's the worst feeling in the world. You literally want to chop your legs off and throw them. You want to take your stomach out and set it down beside you. Your whole body aches, it hurts. You can't move. You're crying, sneezing, you're sneezing and sneezing and sneezing. Your nose is sliding out. Your eyes are watering, they're itchy and you can't stop, and your ears hurt, your head aches, your stomach's cramping. Everything's hard. It's the worst feeling in the world.

Laura (WF33) was right. I don't truly understand and hopefully never will, but it becomes easier to comprehend how your life might start to fall apart if you're preoccupied with avoiding the feeling of wanting to remove your own stomach. Suddenly, making it to work on time or the thought of getting caught stealing from a big-box store doesn't carry the same importance as it used to. You have a new number one, looming so large that there isn't room on your list for anything else. Often, there are no lines that someone in active addiction will refuse to cross. Prior moral and ethical dictums slowly fade away, one by one, until there's nothing left.

Introduction

Since 1980, the number of drug poisoning deaths in the United States has increased ten-fold, rising from 6,100 per year to 67,367 in 2018 (Centers for Disease Control and Prevention, 2020). A substantial proportion of these deaths are attributable to prescription opioid misuse and street opioids like heroin and fentanyl, producing statistically significant increases in deaths amongst males, females, Whites, Blacks, and most age groups (Rudd et al. 2016). While these figures are staggering, considering overdose deaths alone does not reflect the true scope of this public health crisis. The CDC has estimated that, for every prescription opioid-related overdose death, which represent only a fraction of all overdose deaths, there are roughly "10 treatment admissions for abuse, 32 emergency department visits for misuse or abuse, 130 people who were abusers or dependent, and 825 non-medical users" (Case and Deaton 2015, p.15080). Further, the White House Council of Economic Advisors (2017) has estimated that the annual value of the lives lost to opioid deaths is $504 billion, 2.8% of our GDP.

In response, policymakers have sought solutions to reduce the number of opioid overdose deaths. However, as overdose figures continue to rise (Hedegaard et al. 2018), the capacity of existing strategies to effect meaningful change remains uncertain. While we know a considerable amount regarding unprecedented increases in opioid overdose deaths (Case and Deaton 2015; Donroe, Socias, and Marshall 2018), the differential geographic impact between rural and urban communities (Lenardson, Gale, and Ziller 2016; Monnat and Rigg 2016; Palombi et al. 2018; Rigg, Monnat, and Chavez 2018), and how it has affected people across the demographic spectrum (Cheng 2012; Monnat 2018; Rudd et al. 2016), we know little regarding the individual-level processes and influences associated with addicts' initiation, escalation, and cessation of opioid use. This book seeks to address this gap.

17

In the midst of what is arguably the worst drug epidemic that the United States has seen, as well as the ongoing War on Drugs, the importance of implementing effective drug policy and enforcement is crucial. On a regulatory level, responses to the epidemic such as the enactment of prescription drug monitoring programs (PDMPs) sought to stem the tide but have been largely ineffective (Brady et al. 2014; Paulozzi, Kilbourne, and Desai 2011). Sweeping actions such as these, absent well-informed perspective of addicts' trajectories, also carry the risk of creating unintended consequences. Additionally, from a legal perspective, conventional thinking might suggest that another avenue of addressing the crisis is through escalations in the threat of justice contact, under the assumption that criminal behavior can be deterred (Andenaes 1974; Becker 1968). However, it may be the case that the consequences that effectively deter the average offender will have varying levels of success when applied to opioid addicts. Specifically, elevated probability of arrest, periods of incarceration, or stricter drug sentencing may not be effective deterrents among addicts, whose chemical dependencies are likely to have compromised their ability to rationally analyze risk versus reward (Ekhtiari, Victor, and Paulus 2017; Saddoris et al. 2015; Tobler et al. 2016).

In contrast, and more closely aligned with a public health perspective, there may be alternative paths towards effectively predicting lessened opioid use. Given the strength of an addict's commitment to their drug of choice, it may be that the impetus to get clean must come from within and is only tangentially influenced by external factors. In fact, cognitive change criminologists might expect this to be the case, believing that the first step towards the cessation of crime stems from an offender's willingness to be open to change or the personal conviction to pursue it (Giordano, Cernkovich, and Rudolph 2002; Paternoster and Bushway 2009). With respect to opioid addicts, an individual may reach a period in their respective trajectory that

18

marks a turning point, characterized by a desire to get clean (De Leon 2000; Kay and Monaghan 2019). Consequently, the detection of such a moment, as well as an analysis of common underlying processes, has the potential to shape policy to conform more closely to the realities of opioid addiction.

This book seeks to better inform the opioid, deterrence, and cognitive change literatures through the use of in-depth interviews, exploring former opioid addicts' perceptions of criminal justice contact and the central motivations driving their respective decisions to desist from using. After discussing my data and methods, in Part I, I delve into the context surrounding the proliferation of opioid abuse, documenting how members of my sample became ensnared in opioid addiction and how their respective trajectories were shaped by changes in opioid regulation and availability. In Part II, I discuss deterrence and rational choice theories and the ways that existing research has applied it to both general crime and addiction. I also introduce research that has sought to understand the extent to which chemical dependencies, and opioid use in particular, can corrupt individuals' state of mind. From this foundation, I present findings detailing how opioid addicts perceive the risk associated with criminal justice contact, the effect that it has on behavior, and how arrest and/or incarceration influences future drug use and crime. Alternatively, in Part III, I discuss criminological theories that hold that individual cognitive change is integral component of the desistance process. With respect to opioid addicts, it may be that changing mental processes more effectively influence the desire to continue opioid use, rather than external repercussions. I then present results that highlight the importance of significant changes in cognitive decision-making as part of the process of desisting from opioid addiction. Finally, in conclusion, I discuss the implications of my findings and also discuss potentially promising avenues for more effective judicial intervention with opioid-addicted

offenders.

Data and Methods

Sample

I interviewed a total of 75 voluntary participants from three Columbus-based locations, 1) an opioid-specific drug court; 2) a reentry services organization; and 3) an inpatient residential treatment program. First, the drug court program offered opioid-related offenders the opportunity to participate in the program with the incentive of a reduction or dismissal of charges as a condition of completion. Members of the program were broken into one of three phases, with elevated phases indicating greater progress in recovery and programming. Seventy-five to 80 percent of members possessed recent lower-level felony charges related to possession or drug-motivated property crimes. Violent offenders were ineligible for the program. Members were screened for court suitability at the time of their arrest, referred to the program docket, and then the determination was made whether to extend them an invitation to the program. The program was also part of a larger coalition of services providers and often acted as a facilitator for the distribution of treatment and/or residential services for its members.

Second, I sampled participants from the reentry organization's opioid-specific inmate drug rehabilitation program. Similar to drug court, opioid offenders were offered the opportunity for participation in the program during the arraignment process. The program was limited to male offenders, who were housed at a local transitional living facility in a designated wing for participants. The program met for group treatment sessions several times per week for roughly three months. Third, I sampled from a women's inpatient residential program that served opioid users, as well as other drug users. The choice for program involvement varied, with some there of their own volition, while others were participants due to judicial requirements. As such, participants' duration of admission varied. Members of each respective program were randomly drug tested several times per week as part of their respective programs.

I visited each of the three locations before the start of or at the end of scheduled meetings and/or programming to solicit participation. I introduced myself as a researcher affiliated with Ohio State University, described the core questions of the project, outlined eligibility and interview-related requirements, informed them of contact information gathering procedures, the duration of the study (roughly an hour to an hour-and-a-half), and that they would receive a $25 grocery gift card as compensation. I also made the effort to stress anonymity, confidentiality, and my personal separation from the justice system and all organizations outside the university. At the initial point of contact, I collected a name and a phone/email where they could be reached. I emphasized that they need not provide me with their full name, but only a name they would respond to when contacted via the phone number or email address provided to schedule the interview. Participants' contact information form was destroyed after the interview took place.

Individuals were eligible to participate if they had at least one prolonged period of opioid addiction, experienced contact with the justice system (e.g., an arrest and/or a period of incarceration) and had at least six months of clean time at the time of the interview. Their period of addiction need not be exclusive to opioids and could include the use of other drugs; however, they had to have considered opioids to be their "main drug of choice." In exceptional cases, participants with less than six months of clean time, but no less than four months, were permitted to participate under the advisement of facility/treatment personnel that deemed the individual to be "ready" or "in a good place" that allowed them to discuss their addiction without presenting a potential harm to themselves and their sobriety.

Roughly 50 percent of drug court participants volunteered to take part in the study after learning of the eligibility criteria and the purpose of the study. In each of the reentry facility's cohorts, at least 90 percent of individuals volunteered to participate. Lastly, nearly all eligible individuals at the in-patient facility volunteered, such that I needed to generate a waiting list to establish a set ordering. Across all interviews, no individuals withdrew from the study during the consent process, nor did any elect to drop out of the study prior to anticipated completion.

Initially, I had plans to interview 50 participants, but was able to obtain additional grant funding after the completion of the first 50. This funding permitted me the resources to interview another 50 participants. Unfortunately, my 75th interview was conducted in mid-March 2020, days before Covid-19-related safety measures began to take effect. Given the clear safety concerns for subjects and myself, interviews were suspended indefinitely and were not resumed. Due to the highly personal nature of the subject matter, I chose not to pursue video interviews with the belief that a video medium would be qualitatively different than the result of prior in-person interviews. Face-to-face interaction was a crucial component of rapport building, but more importantly, bodily cues, such as subtle changes in vocal inflection or posture, were important indicators of changes in participants' comfort level when discussing a given topic. Nevertheless, I was able to achieve overall saturation on core emergent themes such that the integrity of the study was uncompromised.

The descriptive statistics presented in Table 2 were collected using a brief demographics-oriented survey. The average participant was 33 years old, with a range of 20 to 51 years old. The gender division of my sample was even between males and females. The racial breakdown of the sample was heavily White (84%). Nevertheless, my sample was relatively representative of overall program demographics. If anything, my sample was more diverse, as I made concerted efforts to approach people of color to participate when the opportunity presented itself in efforts to collect data reflecting a diversity of experiences. While often portrayed as such, the opioid epidemic is not just a White problem. In fact, the effects are equally felt by other racial groups (Rudd et al. 2016). As we know, people of color, especially African Americans, are increasingly likely to experience criminal justice-related discrimination (Alexander 2012; Berger 2014; Murakawa and Beckett 2010). Given this reality, and the subjective nature of program admittance, it may be the case that racial demographics influence selection. Admittance is often dependent upon the severity of the crime committed by the offender, with more serious offenders being sorted out. This selection mechanism also poses a potential juncture where discrimination might occur; though, answering these questions falls beyond the scope of this study.

Nearly half of participants were single and roughly 40 percent were in either committed relationships or were married. Participants were also unlikely to receive any form of government aid beyond food stamps, which 59 percent received. A little over half of the sample possessed a high school degree/equivalency or less, while the remainder reported taking some form of college classes, with roughly 10 percent receiving a degree.

At the time of their respective interviews, only 36 percent of the sample was employed. In certain instances, this was not by choice. Depending on program and/or facility rules, it may have been that individuals were discouraged or prohibited from maintaining employment due to programming restrictions. Though, overall, participants reported promising employment prospects. Eighty-eight percent of the sample maintained that, throughout the entirety of their stretches of addiction, they would have been able to find work if they chose to, demonstrating ample opportunity for employment, counter to speculation regarding the negative influence of economic anxiety (Dasgupta, Beletsky, and Ciccarone 2018; Ghertner and Groves 2018; Hollingsworth, Ruhm, and Simon 2017).

The average age of an individual at the time of their first period of addiction was 22 years old. Sadly, some members of the sample reported addictions beginning as early as ten or eleven. Conversely, several adults reported experiencing their first fight with addiction well into their forties, with the oldest being 51 years old. Often, these individuals had no prior problems with substances, but became dependent upon prescription opioids.

On average, an individual in my sample experienced nearly seven separate periods of addiction. This fact is important because it helps address a potential limitation of my sample. Given that most offenders that are offered treatment tend to have less lengthy-criminal records, or may even be first-time offenders, there is a chance that my sample may not have experienced addiction or a criminal lifestyle to the extent that individuals with greater justice contact would have. While a valid concern, it proved to not be the case here. Participants often reported extensive addiction histories preceding any form of contact with the justice system, entailing substantial personal strife and, at times, surprisingly prolific criminal pasts. In this sense, it is naïve to equate membership in what might be seen as a softer diversionary justice program with lesser severity of addiction.

Additionally, participants' several experiences with the cycle of addiction provided ample opportunity for self-reflection. After many successes, followed by a near-equal number of failures, participants were well-positioned to describe the most salient factors that contributed to the ups and downs of their substance use and their state of mind throughout these periods. As part of the desistance process, on average, individuals reported attending nearly four separate treatment or rehabilitation programs, excluding their current programming. Though, participation was not often associated with completion, with individuals only completing an average of 57 percent of the programs they began.

Participants' were 21 years'-old, on average, when they had their first contact with the justice system. Similar to the wide range among members' age at first addiction, individuals that came from especially disadvantaged and troubled backgrounds were first arrested as early as age 10. In the year preceding our interview, the participants were arrested an average of just over one time. Over the course of their lives, participants were arrested an average of nearly 15 times. This figure was influenced by a small handful of offenders that reported a significant number of arrests (50+). More appropriately, and still quite meaningfully, the median participant was arrested seven times.

Beyond an arrest, nearly every person I interviewed had spent time incarcerated. Interestingly, over 70 percent of participants agreed that they would characterize their period(s) of incarceration as "mostly short stays in jail," demonstrating the largely lower level of punishment they experienced as drug offenders. Lastly, it was clear that opioids had a substantial influence on individuals' criminality. On average, participants believed that roughly 85 percent of their lifetime arrests were for drug-defined crimes (e.g., possession, sale) or drug-related-crimes (e.g., property crime to generate funds for drugs).

Many individuals' paths to addiction were intimately tied to a doctor's office. Nearly 80 percent of my sample received an opioid painkiller prescription from a doctor for the treatment of a personal ailment. Of those individuals, nearly 80 percent reported seeking refills early under false pretenses (e.g., dropped them, spilled them down the drain, etc.) and nearly 85 percent reported selling some portion of their own prescription on occasion. Participants often detailed how pills were used as a form of currency, whereby they would sell some to generate cash for immediate needs and would then likely seek to replenish their stash from other sources when finances permitted.

Addicts often had several addiction-relate d medical emergencies, requiring an average of 4.65 trips to the emergency room and/or calls for paramedics. On the more severe end of that spectrum, two-thirds of my sample reported having what they regarded as an "official" overdose. In these instances, legitimacy was individually and subjectively determined. Some conditions for meeting this burden included receiving emergency treatment, the administration of Narcan, etc. Although not captured among this roughly two-thirds portion of the sample, many individuals discussed a tiered perception of overdoses. For example, a given individual may have experienced a loss of consciousness or blacked out while using, but they did not regard the event as a "true" overdose. Conversely, another individual might deem the same event to be an overdose in their personal experience. Accordingly, I allowed the participant to respond to the question using their personal sense of what they believed was an overdose. Ultimately, I believe that the true overdose figure is greater than two-thirds. Based on several participants' re-telling of traumatic incidents, most often related to IV heroin or fentanyl use, individuals that reported never overdosing in the survey portion of the study preceding the interview described circumstances that, while not personally regarded as an overdose, would likely meet most objective criteria for the event. Among the two-thirds of the sample that reported an overdose, it was infrequently an isolated event. On average, those that reported having at least one overdose reported nearly five separate overdoses, many of which resulted in temporary, several-minutes-long deaths.

A large portion of individuals (90.67%) began using opioids through legal or illicitly obtained prescription pills. In either case, the proportion of pill users that eventually transitioned to heroin was staggering. Just over 80 percent of my entire sample transitioned from pills to heroin, with the majority eventually progressing to intravenous use. It was exceptionally rare that an addict only used pills throughout the entirety of their addiction; only four percent did. Conversely, it was equally rare for an addict to bypass pills entirely and go straight to heroin use, with only roughly three percent doing so.

Interviews

I conducted in-depth interviews with 75 former opioid addicts with the goal of gaining a better understanding of the circumstances surrounding their periods of active use, including the initiation, escalation, and cessation of opioid use. Prior to the interview, I gathered demographic data through a researcher-administered survey, lasting roughly five minutes. Data collection began in late November of 2019, continuing until mid-March of 2020. On average, the recorded interviews lasted roughly 80 minutes. Audio files were transcribed prior to coding and were deidentified to ensure anonymity.

Consent was obtained before any activities began. During the consent form review, I made it clear that we would be discussing periods of addiction in considerable detail. We went through the consent form deliberately and I answered any questions ahead of beginning the study, so as to best help individuals decide if participation was in their best interest or might cause them undue stress. No participants withdrew for this reason, nor were any interviews ended prematurely due to participant distress. Participants had full discretion over what subjects were discussed, were advised of their ability to bypass any content, and their ability to leave at any time while still receiving compensation. All interviews took place in a private and separate setting, typically in an empty office or conference room.

My interview guide (included as Appendix A) conformed to Esterberg's (2002) model for semi-structured interviewing and relied upon a set of core questions but also allowed for additional probing questions, which proved especially important given the propensity for addiction to affect the entirety of a person's life. This method gave me the flexibility to discuss each of the core themes in my interview guide, but in an organic fashion that encouraged participants to follow personal lines of thought. This process aided in building rapport with participants, encouraged the use of greater detail, and produced content permitting a deeper assessment of meaning. It also allowed me to delicately navigate topics or experiences that I perceived as being sensitive for the participant. Examples of questions (and probes) include: Can you describe the time when you first used opioids? (How were you introduced to them? What was going on in your life around this time?), In your mind, were there different stages of your use? (What was behind changes in how much you used or how you used?), When you were in your addiction, were you ever worried about being arrested? (Why? How did you think about the prospect of serving time?), How has/have your arrest(s) influenced your drug use? (Have you reduced or stopped using? Increased? Did it take multiple arrests to change things?).

Rapport-building was also likely aided by the demographic make-up of my sample. Given that my sample was 84 percent white and was often young, my status as a 30-year-old White male may have generated an elevated level of comfort among my participants, facilitating candor. While anecdotal, I found that it was common for participants across demographic categories to remark that they were divulging information or sharing experiences that they had previously not disclosed to others, which helped to alleviate my personal concerns regarding positionality during the data collection stage. Throughout the entirety of the research process, I made efforts to authentically emphasize that I was undertaking this project because the opioid epidemic was an issue that I was passionate about and that my focus was on generating insights that could help the "system" better aid individuals in similar positions by learning from their experiences; ultimately, a goal that I would not be able to accomplish without their help.

Coding

I coded interview transcripts concurrent with data collection. This process gave me the opportunity to iteratively revise both my interview guide and coding structure to enhance focus on emerging themes. I followed standard procedures for qualitative analysis of in-depth interview data and used NVivo software to code the data. Codes were refined and amended through an iterative process, approaching the data through multiple readings, coding, and assessing emerging concepts and themes relevant to my research questions (Rubin and Rubin 2012). Although changes were often small, added emphasis on certain sets of probing questions focused on consistent themes (e.g., different perceptions of arrests) in order to gather additional contextual information as well as assess deeper feelings and motivations surrounding events.

Interviews were coded using a combination of inductive and deductive perspectives (Corbin and Strauss 2014). I applied deductive approaches, making theoretically sensitive coding an important component for my main codes, which often corresponded to major criminological theoretical perspectives, including Strain theory (Merton 1938; Messner and Rosenfeld 1994), Deterrence theory (Becker 1968; Stafford and Warr 1993), Control theory (Gottfredson and Hirschi 1990; Hirschi and Gottfredson 1983), Life course theory (Laub and Sampson 1993, 2003; Uggen 2000), and Cognitive change theory (Giordano et al. 2002; Paternoster and Bushway 2009; Skardhamar and Savolainen 2014). Codes also documented certain relevant activities, such as involvement in crime or patterns of drug use. Not all of these codes were utilized in this analysis.

Axial codes sought to efficiently categorize individuals' responses in order to expedite manuscript preparation, given the length and quantity of interviews. For example, under my Deterrence theory main header, a parent node was "Prospect of Incarceration," with child nodes of "Not scared," "Scared, changed behavior," and "Scared, no change in behavior." Over the course of the first 15 readings, child nodes were amended in order to better capture emerging trends. For example, originally, and prior to beginning interviews, child nodes for "Prospect of Incarceration" were simply "Not scared" and "Scared."

Terms and Notation

Throughout the manuscript, I use the terms "addict" and "user" in a variety of situations and variations. In the substance use literature, the term "Person who uses drugs" has begun to supplant those terms; however, I do not use that convention here. My sample exclusively used both "addict" and "user" when describing both themselves as well as other drug users, therefore, I chose to use those terms here in an effort to maintain the authenticity of my participants' portrayals of their lived experiences. As well, in keeping with these efforts, Table 1 provides definitions of slang terms that respondents frequently utilized.

As well, when quotations are introduced, respondents' names are followed by (in parentheses) their race, gender, and age. For example, one participant, John (WM36), is a White male who is 36 years' old. Other shorthand utilized includes B (Black), M (multi-racial), A (Asian), AI (American Indian), and F (female). Transgender individuals' stated gender identity was preceded by a "T." No members of my sample identified as non-binary.

Importantly, the make-up of my sample poses limitations. All participants in my sample were heavy opioid users and were often heroin users. It is important to emphasize that these individuals are outliers regarding their opioid use. While the opioid epidemic is inextricably tied to prescription painkillers, there were millions of individuals that received the pills, used them as directed, and then went about their lives. Even among individuals that misused the pills, the vast majority did not pursue the habit to the extent that the majority of my sample did, stopping well short of heroin addiction. While I present detailed accounts of my participants' addictions and how they unfolded, it is with the recognition that their experiences are atypical and are not representative of opioid users in a general sense. Nevertheless, an examination of the circumstances surrounding their addictions provides important insight regarding the development of advanced opioid use.

Another limitation of my sample selection relates to participants' legal histories. As a criterion for eligibility, a participant must have had some form of contact with the justice system. However, I would contend that opioid addiction and the commission of crime are interconnected in a far greater sense than we typically recognize. The vast majority of my sample had no prior significant criminal past before they became addicted to opioids. So, officially, these individuals weren't criminals up until the point that they were caught for the first time; though, their criminal activity preceding that point in time could typically be described as prolific. As addiction severity increased, especially in the context of the period marking the transition from plentiful pills to relative scarcity, financial hardships accumulated quickly. While monetary resources abated, physiological demand for the drugs increased, triggering elevated levels of desperation to sate cravings. Consequently, addicts turned to crime. Indeed, members of my sample reported that roughly 85 percent of their lifetime arrests were drug-related or directly motivated by the

need to acquire funds to purchase drugs. My sample's median lifetime arrests was also seven.

Table 2: Descriptive Statistics

	Percentage or Mean (St. Dev.)
Age	33.61 (6.73)
Gender	
Male	49.33%
Female	49.33%
Other	1.33%
Race	
White	84.00%
Black	8.00%
Other	8.00%
Relationships	
Single	46.67%
In a committed relationship	37.33%
Married	5.33%
Divorced or separated	10.67%
Number of children	2.12 (1.54)
Social assistance	
Unemployment	2.66%
Disability	0%
Food	58.66%
Highest level of education	
Less than high school	22.67%
High school graduate or GED	34.67%
Some college	40.00%
College graduate or greater	2.67%
Currently employed	36.00%
Able to find work in past and present if desired	88.00%

Continued

Table 2: Descriptive Statistics, Continued

Age at first addiction	22.20 (6.86)
Separate periods of opioid addiction	6.78 (8.21)
Number of rehab visits	3.68 (4.52)
Individual rehab completion percentage	57.17%
Age at first conviction	21.16 (7.51)
Arrests in past year	1.32 (1.60)
Lifetime arrests	14.69 (22.02)
Ever incarcerated	94.66%
Percentage that characterized incarcerations as "mostly short stays in jail"	73.24%

Individual percentage of lifetime
    arrests that were drug- related or drug-
    involved?
	84.78%

Received personal opioid prescription	78.67%
Attempted to get refills early	77.97%
Ever sold personal prescription	84.75%
Instances requiring emergency services	4.65 (8.13)
Ever overdosed	66.67%
Number of overdoses	4.91 (3.51)
Opioids used during active addiction	
Prescription pills	90.67%
Heroin	89.33%
Fentanyl	61.33%

Continued

Table 2: Descriptive Statistics, Continued

Pills only	4.00%
Pills to heroin	81.33%
Heroin only	2.67%
Sampling location	
Drug court	33.33%
Reentry/transitional living treatment	41.33%
Inpatient residential treatment	25.33%

Part I: Where it Started and Where it Led: How Macro-level Shifts Influenced Individual Opioid Use

Most often, efforts to uncover the underlying causes of the explosion of drug and opioid overdose deaths stem from changes in the regulation and prescription of opioid analgesics. In the latter half of the 1990s, The Federation of State Medical Boards released the report "Model Guidelines for the Use of Controlled Substances for the Treatment of Pain," advocating for the "safe and effective treatment of patients with pain, including…the use of opioid analgesics"(Federation of State Medical Boards of the United States, Inc. 1998). While likely well-intentioned, and certainly meant to treat patients suffering from chronic pain, the report established a questionable mandate that resulted in the proliferation of opioid analgesics with deleterious results (Lembke 2016). On the heels of new, looser regulations, prescription sales exploded. From 1997 to 2002, Oxycodone, methadone, and fentanyl sales increased 402.9, 410.8, and 226.7 percent, respectively (Paulozzi 2006). Furthermore, national sales have maintained this elevated trajectory to the present, quadrupling since 1999. Consequently, these drugs became more accessible to the average person, both legally and illegally, resulting in mirrored increases between opioid distribution and overdose deaths (Rudd et al. 2016). What makes the increase in opioid distribution more troubling is that efforts to regulate consumption have largely been ineffective. Prescription drug monitoring programs were not significantly associated with lower rates of overdose, overdose mortality, or rates of opioid consumption (Brady et al. 2014; Paulozzi et al. 2011) or were only associated with modest overdose death reductions in others (Johnson et al. 2014; Rutkow et al. 2015). In the midst of increased regulatory attention to the problem at hand, it begs the question– "Why are people still continuously dying at such high rates?"

In many ways, opioid addiction can be traced back to the proliferation of pills. Just over 91 percent of my sample entered opioid use through prescription painkillers. Whether the pills are prescribed to a person, their mother, or someone that drove down to Florida to get a bogus MRI and the hook-up, it doesn't change what the pills are. Regardless of how someone is exposed to them, painkillers are highly addictive, but what makes them especially dangerous is how they are perceived (Remillard, Kaye, and McAnally 2019). In the eyes of many, painkillers are medicine that comes from a doctor and because it comes from a doctor, they're not really drugs (Daniulaityte, Falck, and Carlson 2012). If you're in pain, just take another. They're medicine. In a sense, the pills get a free pass from scrutiny. Before popular discourse began to recognize the harmful effects that they carried, hundreds of thousands of individuals developed addictions to them, the consequences of which have been far-reaching.

The changing landscape of pain pill regulation has dictated shifts in opioid use in fundamental ways. When prescription pain pills flooded the drug market, they were dirt cheap. Only when government agencies began to become aware of how the system was being played did change occur. By then, it was too late. What was once so abundant that it was handed out to friends like candy on Halloween had become a highly-regulated commodity in what felt like a blink of the eye (Kelly, Vuolo, and Marin 2017). Individuals that had become physically dependent on opioids no longer had a source. Whether they were receiving their own script, buying them off the street, or both, the game was over, and they were dope sick. Whatever pills addicts could find were far too expensive. Not that it really mattered anyway. For users with several years of built-up tolerance, just finding enough to get well was a fanciful notion. If by some miracle they could, the prospect of spending upwards of $600 in a day placed them well beyond reach. Sick and desperate, addicts had a choice to make, and it was not going to entail riding out withdrawals.

While the individuals in my sample came from divergent backgrounds and entered pill use in myriad ways, over 80 percent of the individuals that used pills ended up using heroin; the vast majority of whom would progress to the final, most damaging stage– intravenous use. There isn't anything specific to the pills that makes them a gateway to heroin use. Even though it's common to quickly develop a tolerance, many prefer to stay on the pills, often strongly so. The transition to heroin carries a stigma. One can no longer think of themselves as a "normal" person. Normal people don't use heroin. Even amongst addicts, heroin users occupy a lowly position in the hierarchy of drug users. But, as the pills dried up, heroin became the go-to. It made sense. It was cheap, was becoming easier to get, and it would last longer. At a certain point, the pro/con calculations of a cash-strapped opioid addict only produced one outcome and there was a strong chance that this moment transpired sometime in the early-to-mid 2010s. So, while there wasn't anything inherent to pill use that preordained heroin use, significant changes in the regulation and availability of pills did.

While we have considerable knowledge related to the magnitude of the pills' proliferation, we know relatively little about how this process unfolded on an individual level (Cicero and Ellis 2017). In the first chapter of this section, I shed light on important questions regarding how contextual factors influenced opioid users' addictions. Namely, I explore how addicts' use was shaped by the seemingly endless supply of pills flowing from the exploitation of a broken medical system and the unforeseen consequences of systemic regulatory reform. In the second, I investigate individuals' perceptions of the pills, unpacking how the drugs' innocuous, and even legitimate status contributed to the growth of peoples' addictions. I then follow this thread, tracking how individuals, some with no prior history of drug use, became full-blown

heroin addicts.

Chapter 1. The Florida Connection: Passengers, Operators, and the Back Door to a Script

"You go down there, get an MRI done, then go back to the doctor with the MRI that says your back's fucked up, and then they give you a massive amount of everything and come back and sell them. They give you enough drugs to fucking kill 20 elephants at once."

- John (WM36)

The worst kept secret on the street in the mid-to-late-2000s involved piling everyone you could find into a van, driving 15 hours, and coming home with thousands of pills. Do it every few weeks and working a straight job becomes optional. The scheme was simple– get down to Florida, get an MRI for "back pain," then take that to a doctor that had a reputation for being loose with their prescription pad (Rigg, March, and Inciardi 2010). The process wasn't hard. In 2010-2011, a small percentage of doctors were writing up to 16 times more opioids prescriptions than the average Florida physician (Chang et al. 2016). Anyone with even a tangential connection to the scheme could give you the names and locations of at least a couple places you could go. Over half of my sample was involved in the scheme in some capacity, demonstrating just how pervasive it was among opioid users. Individuals with jobs, families, and no prior ties to drug use or crime knew about it and often became wrapped up in it. Pill mill activity wasn't limited to a certain socioeconomic bracket. If you were using opioids post-2005, you knew about Florida.

Passengers: The Exploitable Desperation of Addicts in Need

Renee (MF32) was a recent entrant into opioid use. She'd been selling weed off and on since she was 20 but never moved much weight. She was small-time. It was just supplementary income that let her actually start a savings off of her minimum wage job. Spend the drug money, save the paychecks. Slender and unassuming, it was hard to imagine that she'd ever done anything illegal in her life. Being involved in that sort of lifestyle, exposure to opioids was a given. She was introduced to them by a close friend. More than anything, she tried them out of curiosity. Everyone around her was doing them. They started out as a fun thing to do at parties, but quickly became more than that, "That's when I started doing opioids…my friend had it one time and I did it and I liked how I felt. And then I'd wait a couple of days and do it again. And then once you do it for so many days in a row, it's over. Seriously, if you do something three or four days in a row after that, you started getting sick from it."

Over the next few weeks, her habit escalated as she tried to keep the symptoms in check and the money she made from selling weed wasn't covering it. She found herself talking to her supplier about how she was starting to feel sick when she didn't have them. She knew he'd been making trips down to Florida, but that was the extent of it. He'd come back with pills, but that wasn't her thing, so she didn't pay any mind to it. But all of the sudden, making the trip herself was starting to sound enticing, "It started off as $500 and 50 pills for free… So, I'm like, 'All right.' At this point, I've never been to Florida before. They pay for the hotel. I will stop at the beach. All your food's paid for. It's a lightweight vacation." What's not to like? A free vacation to a place you'd never been, money, and pills. The first trip down went smoothly, so she kept going, each time bringing back a bounty of pharmaceuticals,

> When I went to Florida, they prescribe everything. They prescribed for Percocet, Xanax bars, and perc 30s, perc 15s. Everyone on the Hilltop [a lower-income Columbus neighborhood] knew about it, so everyone was going down there. People would take vans of people. The doctor's offices were crowded...There were a few facilities. Everyone went to Hope4Life in Miami. There's one in Fort Lauderdale, it was really crooked. Our pharmacy technician saying so. Thinking

back, we would give all of our prescriptions to one guy and he would go to Walgreens before it even opened and the pharmacist would fill all of our stuff and he'd come back with all of it. I'm like, "How the fuck?"

The Sunshine State had become a veritable Candyland. A quick three-day, two-night trip and you came back with more pills than you'd need in three months for something a few Advil could probably handle. In Renee's case, she was perfectly healthy. No accidents, no injuries. It didn't matter. Going through the motions was just a perfunctory thing. In certain clinics, there was no such thing as a clean MRI. Anyone and everyone that came through the doors was in excruciating pain and in dire need of medication.

Given the moneymaking potential, it's not surprising that going down to Florida quickly became a well-orchestrated operation for many. As the practice grew, people from Ohio found themselves integrated into the operation at all different levels. Like Renee, many remained at the lowest level– they were passengers, just along for the ride.

Gary (WM31) was one of those people. Gary had a rough life. He'd lived on the streets off and on his entire life and it showed. Most prominent was the long indent running down the length of the middle of his forehead, a result of the collapse of his "favorite vein" from over a decade of IV drug use. He'd come from an unstable home where his father was a trucker and wasn't around much. When he was, he wasn't exactly the best influence. Two weekends a month, seven-year-old Gary and his dad would watch porn and drink beers while his mom was at work. There were even times where his dad would let him do a line of coke if he felt like sharing. Gary's odds of becoming an upstanding member of society were always low and it wasn't his fault. In the end, he just continued to do what his family had modeled to him as normative.

He first got in trouble at ten when he got caught in the principal's office with an ounce of weed in his pants, this while he was in the office for fighting. Trouble followed him wherever he went, even across the country when he was sent off to live with an uncle in order to give him a fresh start. Right off the bus to a far-away state, he was drawn to an individual wearing a trench coat, lined with pockets filled with just about every drug you could imagine. Life continued on that track, becoming a father at 17 and hustling to make whatever money he had.

Part of living a hustler's lifestyle meant being exposed to danger. Gary had been shot, stabbed, and beaten within an inch of his life more than once over drugs. While it didn't deter him from continuing as he always had, it did make him an ideal candidate for clinic visits in Florida. With so many significant injuries, including a crushed vertebra, multiple skull fractures, and a traumatic brain injury (TBI), his MRIs were guaranteed to "come back good." "I worked for a dude that he'd take three vans, like caravans, and fill them up with all kinds of people. TBI, you know what I mean? I got a lot of injuries in my life, so I'll go down there, and we'd find a bunch of people like me and he'd pay us. We'd go down there and get the scripts and fill them. He'd give me cash." Not only would his "employer" have three full vans that regularly made the trips, but all 30+ of them would then recruit as many indigent individuals as they could in order to maximize the number of pills they could get, generating over $150,000 worth of pills in a single trip.

Like Gary, Liz (AF34) viewed being a passenger on Florida trips as easy money. At the time, it was exactly what she needed. From age 17, Liz had always worked in clubs. She started by taking drink orders and cleaning up. When she turned 18, she started dancing and was making around $500 per night. She hated school and making so much money meant she could stop going. She'd used before, and liked it, but it was only a pill here or there. Having the income from the club meant that she had money to spend. Combined with the type of environment she worked in, the increase in her drug use just sort of happened, "I worked at strip clubs and stuff like that to feed my drug habit because, of course, even though I wasn't addicted, I still like to do drugs and that paid for my way." Paying for drugs with money that she didn't really need expedited her addiction. She maintains that between 18 and 23 she wasn't addicted, but, regardless of personal labels, she was starting to use daily not long after she started dancing. A bouncer she knew at the club always had a Ziploc full of pills of different shapes and colors, so getting them was as convenient as could be. With such easy access, she slowly worked her way up the opioid ladder. She started with perc 5s or vike 5s (Vicodin), going up to perc 15s when she really wanted to feel it, and then to perc 30s and/or Oxy 80s (OxyContin) when the 15s weren't really doing anything anymore. Only three months after her first exposure, she was up to 13 perc 30s per day. She'd also begun shooting the pills rather than snorting or eating them, marking a significant progression in her use.

Her burgeoning addiction had excised her from the inheritance left by her grandparents when they passed. The abusive relationship she had with her mother meant that her grandparents were a stand-in for her lack of a relationship with her own parents. She was distraught when they died, but more pressingly, her immediate situation became dire quickly. Her grandparents had always given her whatever she wanted, including considerable sums of money whenever she asked. Now, her enablers were no longer alive and her cut of the $150,000 they left behind was a $500 shopping spree at Walmart. Suddenly, she needed every dollar that she made at the club. Her opioid dependence was no longer aligned with her financial capabilities and that meant she was getting sick. There wasn't anyone to bail her out. Now, unable to spend her entire night's pay on pills, she had to get creative.

When a friend at the club told her about Florida, she was eager to go. They referred her to someone they knew and that was that. They handled everything. All she had to do was show up,

> They would doctor shop. I would go down, get a script for the 30s. If they had to, they pay to get the script filled. Then I give them the pills and they give me like $200, but they were making like $2,000 off of a bottle of pills…I'd go as often as I could. Probably about four times a month if not more. Pay the doctor if I needed to for him to write the script. Go get the script filled. I got a couple of pills out of it and so the person that took us down, he bought the script off of us. It was legit. It was just not right, I mean. If that makes any kind of sense. It was legally. They could ask the doctor, 'Did they write a script,' and doctor says, 'Yeah.' In my part, it was legit; but on that side, maybe it wasn't…I would just go to my doctor's appointments every month and get my script.

Liz's only responsibility was to go to her appointments. The operators knew where to go and who to pay. Liz had become part of a well-oiled machine. She needed the money, so she was thankful, but she knew she was being taken advantage of. It just didn't bother her. She was content with earning around $1,000 a month for doing nothing other than escaping grey, dreary Ohio days. She knew that whatever they were doing to organize it all was shady at best and likely illegal, and she didn't want any part of that.

Like Liz, others started to catch on to what was happening– they were getting ripped off. Operators fronted travel expenses and would buy the scripts off them, but for pennies on the dollar. As pill addicts, they were well-versed in the drug market and knew how much pills cost at any given time. After only a trip or two, the math was easy to do. A few hundred dollars for pills with a cumulative street value of around $5,000 didn't seem like as good of a deal once the pills are actually in your hands. The choice then became to either continue as a passenger for larger-scale operators, like Liz, or to branch off on your own and start a personal scheme.

Keisha (MF38) was a veteran Florida passenger before she started her own thing. She'd been making the trips a few times a month for years and knew the ins and outs of the operation better than most. She'd been using for decades, so she was hip to the scheme from the beginning. Keisha got into drugs young. She started sneaking alcohol around 12 and was a full-blown opioid addict at 16. She was born to a 16-year-old mother who was always in trouble. Her mother was White and her father Black. He was never involved in her life and the two never met. Living in rural West Virginia, having a Mixed child meant Keisha's mother, already a single mother, would endure constant racist taunts, "they forbid the black and white mingling, so she pretty much got ran out of West Virginia." After leaving what little family they had behind, the two moved around frequently, rarely staying in one place more than a few months. Things never got better. Most of what Keisha remembers of her childhood revolves around her mother's erratic behavior, "I remember my mom drinking. I remember my mom using drugs. She still uses drugs up to now. Lots of domestic violence, a lot of her going to jail." Her mom was in and out of jail until the time Keisha turned 18, but Keisha had been an adult well before then. At 14, she started running away from home for extended periods of time. She dropped out of school in the ninth grade and started hustling to make money. With no one around, she could do whatever she wanted and that became drugs, dabbling in everything from weed, to coke, to pills.

In her early 20s, Keisha was able to leave that life behind. She had a daughter, and everything fell into place, that was, until the accidents. A few years later, Keisha was in a series of car accidents. Five in one year. She was in the passenger seat for the first one, so severe that she had to be life flighted to a nearby hospital. She survived, but severe anxiety attacks meant she wouldn't drive herself after. Then came the other four, all as a passenger. With each accident, her body was developing new aches and pains from the cumulative trauma and the several surgeries she'd needed. Each time she was in the hospital they'd give her something for the pain and send her off with a script. While she was hospitalized, they were consistently giving her perc 30s to help manage the pain. For someone else, this may not have been a problem, but Keisha's history of addiction meant that having the pills was like opening a door to the past.

> I'm leaving and they gave me 5s. I called back and said, "Hey, the 5s aren't working." They wouldn't tell me to bring the 5s in and get another prescription. So, I was taking them. I was abusing them. Going to different doctors, going to emergency rooms. They told me to come and get a prescription because they really were trying to see where my pain level was because I was in a hospital. And they was giving me 30s in there so they couldn't just take me off…I would come home on 5s and I would wait a day or two and I would say, "This pain is not gone..." They'd say, "Okay come get a prescription for 10s." Cause they're really trying to find out what's my pain type. So as long as I keep saying they're not working, they're keep going up, so I learned that. And then my urine was always clear, only had the pill in there. So, the doctor was saying, "Well she is taking them," but he didn't know that I was abusing them.

Keisha figured out how to game the system quickly. Even though her pain was legitimate in the beginning, her prior addiction to opioids left her vulnerable to abusing them. As soon as she had them in the hospital, it was like something "woke up" in her. She craved them again. From that point, it was a slippery slope back to exactly where she'd left off years prior, and then beyond. She was careful to not use any other drugs in order to ensure she passed any drug tests, but she was also able to take advantage of a system that lacked inter-doctor communication or a centralized prescription monitoring database. On paper, she was only prescribed perc 10s, but she was getting them from several locations, allowing her to effectively take several 30 milligram doses in the course of a day.

During prior periods of use, she was always able to get what she needed. There was never a prolonged period where she went without and experienced sickness. After 16 months, her doctors began to put the pieces together. She was getting sloppy managing the doctors. As her physical need grew, she pushed them too hard and they cut her off. What followed was a new experience for her, "I never went without them. And I really thought, "'Okay, it was just fun. I'm having fun, I've got pills, I'm not sick.' I never knew that about being sick because I didn't go without. But when I did get off that pill, the way I felt I knew I had a problem." She couldn't afford to buy them off the street and she was in a position where her dependence was beyond the point where she thought she could stop cold turkey, so like Liz, Keisha started to put out feelers to figure out how to solve her predicament, "they said no [the doctors]. And I found somebody that was going out of town. So, I hopped on that." Keisha had burned bridges at most local medical sources, so the ability to travel out of state was exactly what she needed. Without any income beyond was she could scrounge up, the concept of getting paid to take a quick vacation and get some free pills was an offer she couldn't refuse. She was perfect for the role, given her extensive injury history. She was guaranteed to pass any MRI checks they might want even if they were legit, making her an attractive passenger to make the trip,

> We were driving to Clearwater, Florida. We went down there to the doctor. I went in, I told him...because I knew I already had an MRI, so I knew the problem. So, I had that...pretty much you just walk in there and tell them and they'll give you a prescription or go get an MRI. You just go to the place that they in cahoots with, get the MRI, and at the doctor appointment the next day it was like, $200 for the first visit. The whole script for 120, $4.00 per pill. We was going down there, he would give us $600– he'll give us $600 when we give him the pills. Because he'll give you a couple pills. It was like, "Hey, $600. Well, I ain't got nothing."

With no money and no prospective income, $600 was a large sum for Keisha. She'd get 15-20 pills and would take the money she got and spend that on pills once she was back in Ohio. From the beginning, she was able to do the math. She knew there was a substantial discrepancy between the pills' value and what she got out of the deal, but she was just fine with that, "Everyone would say, 'Oh he's getting over on you because you know he'll get paid $30 for selling them.' He's got to provide transportation. He pays for the food, he's got to pay for the visit, the pills, and everything. So, $600 for just going to the doctors, it seemed like, good at the time."

Staying at the passenger level was attractive because, in her eyes, it involved significantly less risk. Technically, what they were doing was legal if they weren't doctor shopping. As a Florida "resident," they were insulated from repercussions as long as they walked the fine line separating safety from greed. They were just Florida residents that spent a lot of time in Ohio. What's wrong with that? Though, walking the line was easier said than done. It was too tempting, too simple. If you're out of pills and broke, Florida was your life raft and the operators running the crews knew it. Strung out and desperate, maintaining a consistent, legal trip schedule was difficult. In Keisha's case, she decided to branch out and found 3 or 4 different operators to take her down. Each operator typically had several different sets of consistent passengers that would rotate weekly, so she made sure she was a part of several crews, none of them knowing about her trips with the other operators. Keisha was crossing over into criminal territory and she knew it, but that was a risk she was willing to take,

> I never really looked at it like the whole time I could've went to jail for a long time. Because we was going to Tampa, Fort Lauderdale, that's pretty much doctor shopping… Me, I went to four places down there each month. I went once a week. And the first week would be Clearwater. Next week- he had different sets

of people. So, every time we went it was people, sets. He had a total of 13 people. He was getting some money…you were going somewhere new. Maybe we'll go to the beach and stuff or we'll spend the night in a nice hotel.

I knew it was wrong when he started saying, "This is your pill, you keep your pills on you. You've got to have your Florida I.D." and stuff like that, so I knew it was a problem. If he gave me the money right now, that means they're his. So yeah you got to keep your pills on you because for DEA can stop you– you allowed to go and get your prescription in Florida. What you're not allowed to do is get pills from Ohio, Florida, Fort Lauderdale, and different places. You're only allowed to get 120 of each milligram. And if you go over that, that's when the DEA come in to play. So, I could get 120 30s, 120 15s, 120 20s, you know if they went over that's when the doctor shopping came. That's what was happening. I was getting 120 times 4 every month. But you know 120 is supposed to last you a month. So yeah– I think it was the addict in me saying it was worth it.

Keisha stuck to this path the entire time she made Florida trips. Getting roughly $3,000 each month for 12 days work was worth it. Both Keisha and Liz could have gotten better deals. There were plenty of operators all over city and there was a good chance that any short bus or panel van in a bad neighborhood was heading south sooner or later. But for both, the existing arrangement was an easy, passive process and that was appealing to them. Conversely, others decided that if they were going to go, they were doing it on their own. If you aren't forced to sell off most of your entire script, you might be able to subsist on one trip's worth for a month and avoid doctor shopping and the risk it carried.

For years, Monique (MF31) had an easy source to get pills. She lived with her grandma, who had been battling a string of severe illnesses for years. For the pain, she was prescribed copious amounts of perc 30s, far more than she'd ever care to use. With the vast majority of the bottle just sitting there, accumulating with each passing month, Monique figured it wouldn't hurt anything to take a few, "I would be planning to go out with friends or something and I would sneak in and steal some of my grandmother's pills to take with me. So, I don't know if at that point if I was stealing them because I needed them or stealing them because I wanted them." Eventually it would, without a doubt, be because she needed them. But sadly, her grandmother passed not long after Monique entered advanced addiction. Her grandma wasn't just the woman that had raised her, she was also Monique's enabler.

Monique had a void that needed filling, making her easily exploitable. Someone she knew that had a crew was aware of her situation and offered her a spot. She jumped at the opportunity, "The first time I went somebody else paid for it. I went with a girlfriend of mine. It was her friend had paid for a bunch of us to go. We all piled in and drove down, got a decent room. We were gone for like, I don't know, three days or something like that." What she didn't realize was how organized the process was.

> It was like clockwork. I had my appointment. I'd be lucky to make it two weeks. Then I would have to buy more to get me through the next two weeks and then do it all over again. It was so stupid. Turn around and sell them and then you have to turn around and spend the money, if not more money. But if I didn't sell them and I held onto them I think I'd get lucky and get like three weeks, and then I would still run out the last week.

Going on runs for operators was just a stopgap. Her use outpaced the cash and the fraction of the script that she got to keep. Going once a month wasn't cutting it,

> A month or two later I started just going on my own. I would either drive down and drive back, or I would fly down and rent a car and fly back. Every month. I was just seeing one doctor. I was legal as far as the State of Florida was concerned. I made myself a resident of Florida with a Florida ID and everything. I'd see a Florida doctor. I wasn't seeing doctors in Ohio or anything like that. The

only part of it that wasn't legal is me bringing them back here to sell. That's how I was able to fly, right? "I'm a Florida resident, I'm getting my medicine. I spend a lot of time in Ohio. So what? Right? People do it all the time. There's no borders." That happened for a couple years.

Where Keisha had solved her problem by working for several operators, Monique chose to solve hers by taking on more responsibility. Rather than doctor shopping with different operators, she chose to make the trips herself and only see one doctor. This way she was able to keep her entire script, enough to last her a month when you combine the pills' milligram values. Her name was still going in a file somewhere, but she was in a position of relatively low risk by going to the same doctor.

Monique's reaction to working as a passenger was much more common than Keisha's. Giving away at least half of your drugs wasn't something that sat well with most addicts, like Paul (WM34). Paul was first exposed to opioids when his car went off the road and into a ravine when he was 17. He injured his neck badly and still has pain whenever it gets colder. Unlike a lot of medical opioid users, Paul was disciplined with his use. He'd take his low dose percs as scheduled, nothing more.

> Looking back on it, I would say that it was habitual then, although not really knowing the end result, that I would be addicted to them. I didn't know, I was just doing it as prescribed. At this time, I wasn't taking more than I was supposed to, blah blah blah. So, what had ended up happening is they weren't having the same effect, you know? I told this to my doctor. I at first told my dad, and he was like, "Yeah, you need to ask them to up your dose." So that progressed from the 5 milligrams to 7.5s.

Over the next few years, he remained on the pills for chronic pain as part of a treatment regimen that also included frequent cortisone shots that enabled him to continue working as a machine operator. Predictably, as his tolerance continued to grow, his doctor slowly upped his dose. At a certain point, Paul started to notice that he felt a bit "off" when he forgot to take one on his regular schedule and that the higher dose pills were doing things for him that smaller ones didn't, "Once I got up to the 15s, I really started noticing like how you would get the symptoms from your face itching and stuff like that, or I don't know. You would get noticeably higher from the 7.5s to the 15s. And that's when I started taking more than I was actually prescribed."

Paul was afforded excellent medical insurance from work. He had low co-pays and they covered everything, including his percs. In a bad turn of luck, he was laid off from his job as part of his employer's staffing cuts. He looked for work, but the process was getting harder as he was starting to encounter pill sickness. When he was let go, he lost his insurance along with his job. Without the pills and any income, he was sick constantly, "I had never experienced withdrawal. Like, my stream was steady. And if I had insurance, I went to work, I had medication. I never experienced the withdrawal until I actually lost the job. I thought I came down with the flu and one of my buddies was, he's like, 'Dude, you've been taking the pills and you haven't had any, right?'" If he was going to find work, he needed to get well. His girlfriend at the time, witnessing his situation firsthand, told him about how some people she knew had been going down to Florida and coming back with loads of percs, so she made the introduction,

> We were going to Florida once a month. And you could go down there, it was like you'd show up at a doctor's office, they'd do a CAT scan there. "Oh, this, this, and this is wrong. Where do you have pain?" You get the same prescription. So, you'd get 240 there. I was getting 30s, I want to say. The guy, he had a big SUV. And he's like, he'll pay for your doctor and give you half of the prescription. All you have to do is go. I mean if you could go down there for basically free, spend a couple of days down there on the beach, whatever. And all he wanted was half the prescription. I would do that…that's at the beginning. I think I only did like two or

three times and then I started going. Because I'm like, man, "I'm giving this dude half my script." I mean, at this time the pills were going for $20.00, $25.00 a piece, and I was getting 240 of them.

With each trip, Paul received roughly $6,000 worth of pills. He'd only come away with around $500 cash and a few pills making the trip for this particular operator. By shifting to going on his own, he would be able to use more than he had previously, and he did. Like Monique, he was careful. He'd only go to one doctor, once a month. He'd go by himself and pay cash, roughly $300, and fill the script at a pharmacy in Florida recommended to him by the doctor's office.

Operators: Making Easy Money Gaming a Broken System

The common denominator among all of the individuals that served as passengers is that, at the time they were making the trip down south, they had all done so out of desperation. Each persons' habit was exceeding what they were able to obtain and working as a passenger for operators became the answer. On the other side of the equation, nothing was done out of desperation. For operators, desperation was something to be leveraged into filling seats in a van to maximize profits. The size of an operator's scheme varied considerably. Some paid people to take down only 3 or 4 passengers at a time. It carried less risk, but it also yielded significantly less reward. Others orchestrated intricate, consistent schemes that were focused on obtaining as many pills as possible to then either sell on the street through their own distribution networks or to wholesale to dealers.

Sam (WM41) was big-time. Over the course of a 4-year period, he was part of an operation that acquired somewhere in the neighborhood of ten million dollars in Florida-prescribed pills. Prior to starting up a Florida crew, Sam had never been involved in anything that even resembled an organized approach to crime. When Sam was younger, he got into his fair share of trouble. Throughout high school he'd cut class and to go smoke weed and drink with his buddies in the woods of their small, rural Ohio town, "just doing all the things in the back road like country guys do." By the time he was 18, he'd dropped out and started working local manual labor jobs, mostly in construction. By virtue of living in a small town, he could go to the bar everyone frequented and be served without a problem. Everybody knew everybody and no one cared. Hanging out in the bar every night ultimately led to predictable outcomes. He was young and curious about other drugs, so when he had the chance to try coke and acid, he wasn't afraid to experiment. He kept working labor jobs for the next few years, but a dirt bike accident put an end to that.

When he was 23, Sam went out in the country riding dirt bikes with friends like he'd done hundreds of times before but took a spill. He landed awkwardly on his elbow and tweaked his neck. He didn't think much of it. A few Tylenol and some rest. He wasn't in a lot of pain, but his neck was still bothering him two days later, so he figured it was time to go to the doctor,

> I actually broke my neck. Felt like a stubbed toe, you know what I mean? It felt like you jam your finger or toe, that's what my neck felt like. Then I went and they strapped me to the bed and told me "Don't move. You'll be paralyzed from the chest just down." It freaked me out. I'm like, "What the hell you talking about?"… I mean my elbow hurt worse than anything from where I pinched the nerve. It's like my elbow was broken or something…I walked around for two days with a broken neck before I went to the hospital…I actually had to wear a halo.

The next two-and-a-half months were challenging for Sam. Even simple things like laying his head on his pillow at night were completely different. He wasn't allowed to shower and had to have family help him take sponge baths and wash his hair. And then there was the pain. He wasn't bothered by the break initially, but that would change. It kept him awake most nights and the pills helped. He'd never tried pills before, so he felt the full effects of the Oxy 80s they gave him, the pill at the top of the opioid food chain.

> I know the whole couple months that they had me on them it took one to knock me out. It was strong as shit and I was never gone before [knocked out]. So, once they just really took the halo and stuff off…they just cut me off. I started withdrawing a little bit from it and I started buying them off the street and sort of self-medicating every time I got pain and it was off to the races it seemed like from there.

Like Paul, Sam's accident was his gateway to opioid use. Neither had ever used pills before they were prescribed to them by their respective doctors and both took them as prescribed before they ever knew what withdrawals were. In Sam's case, he had the money to be able to buy them off the street. He knew who to go see. Doing coke off and on for the past few years meant he "had a guy." After nearly three months of bed rest, he was itching to get back to work. Between the sickness and the pain, he was frequently buying pills to stay well and to be able to work.

> When I was taking the meds, I didn't feel nothing. [after stopping] I'd feel a lot of aches and pains, yeah. I had a crushed vertebra, it's not like they straightened it back out. It's still crushed and cracked in a couple places…I just took them. My mom came to stay with me, so I mean she always came over and made sure...she lived right next door, so she'd come over and she always gave me the pills when I needed them. So, I wasn't abusing them then, it's after the prescriptions ran out and I started back to work and then I started getting aches and pains, then I started buying them off the street and self-medicating because I didn't have insurance or nothing. I never really realized about the problem, I just thought it was like a leisure thing, you know what I mean? I did it more for the buzz of it, then after a while I kind of just...I started my mind away from the pain and I started taking

> them because I liked the way it made me feel. It just progressed from there. And
> then I started going to Florida, doing the Florida pill runs.

Sam's injury wasn't something that would heal up and he'd be back to normal. He was in a position where he was looking at chronic pain issues for the foreseeable future. Even worse, Sam had reached the point where the pills served a dual purpose– his pain would subside, but they also gave him a new, better normal. Without insurance, he wasn't able to go see a doctor or get refills, so getting them off the street was really Sam's only option, especially after he'd crossed into using them for pleasure. Doctor shopping to places outside his small town wasn't something that ever crossed his mind, that was, until someone told him about Florida.

Without a high school diploma or a GED, labor jobs were Sam's go-to. He swore he wouldn't work fast food and his neck was making construction nearly impossible, even on the pills. In his mind, the next logical move was to start selling them. He'd worked his way up from the 5s and 10s he was buying off the streets to perc 30s, lots of them. Now that he was selling, supply wasn't a problem. He was making good money, but not having a 9-to-5 job made things worse. With nothing to do all day, he just ate pills,

> It's only when I progressed and started getting on the 30s and stuff like that every
> day is when I noticed, like really noticed like the physical sensations and couldn't
> move and the nausea and the hot and cold flashes. That's when I really noticed
> because I quit working and I started selling them. When I was selling them, I was
> doing more of them, a lot more of them because I'm sitting there not doing nothing
> but selling drugs. I'm sitting there just shoveling them in.

Shoveling drugs is going to increase the severity of your dependence, and he was starting to realize it. Though, at the time, the boredom was the bigger problem. He had loads of pills, but also added crack and meth to the mix and would spend weeks at a time partying and selling. The pills were mostly something for maintenance, but he'd use them heavily when he wanted to come down after using stimulants. Up until this point, Sam was a middleman. He'd get the pills from a supplier and sell them, typically to people that he knew in order to minimize his exposure.

After learning about Florida, Sam and some friends became part of a larger network making coordinated pill runs. He had pre-existing connections that gave him an entry point. At first, they were just drivers– paid around $5,000 take others down to the clinics for a larger operator. While they were making the trips, they saw firsthand how many pills passengers were being prescribed, and, having a familiarity of the pills' street value, recognized the opportunity. Before branching off on their own, they started going to the clinics themselves while they were driving for operators and sold the pills they were given when they got home. It gave them knowledge that they'd then use to instruct their own passengers on how to conduct themselves. Sticking as a driver was less risk, but he and his friends recognized an opportunity that was too good to pass up, so they went into business for themselves,

> I got together with some friends. You can get MRIs cheap. So, I went down there with some money and got the MRI done. Went to see the doctor and he prescribed me I think it was like 210 perc 30s; 100 perc 15s. I never doctor shopped, I just went down there once a month, but I took other people down…We're paying for all them to get their shit done, but we're getting their script and then I can sell their scripts too. I was going down there at least twice a month for probably four years straight at least two, sometimes three times a month. It was a pretty big revenue money coming in. Most of them was always getting about 200 or so 30s. So, we'd give them so many of the percs and when they were done, "You want some of the pills or do you want some money?" A lot of times they'll take the money and lots of times they took the pills too, it just depends. Once they got the money then they started getting up on the pills themselves. It was like you was getting all that back anyway. We'd take down probably 20 people or so, we had a bus.

Their experience working for other operators gave them insight into how best approach

compensation– offer them a small number of pills or slightly more cash. The passengers would

take the cash, turn around, and buy some pills back from them just below street value. Do it this

way, and paying passengers became a fraction of their overhead. No longer having to pay

suppliers, he and his crew were starting to make serious money.

While incredibly profitable, the stress associated with running an operation of his own

was getting to Sam. Driving a bus of 20+ people to illegally doctor shop will do that. He was

using a high volume of perc 30s months prior, but the added stress drove him to ramp up his use

to cope with the anxiety,

> I started using more on the trips. It seemed that's when I started using like a lot
> heavier. That's when I progressed where I use a little bit just to kind of mellow me
> out and get my racing thoughts and anxiety under control. So, it kind of
> progressed from there. I'll get high real quick and numb that feeling and I won't be
> fucking more paranoid. It just made me use more. There for a while I was doing
> probably 40 30s a day.

Getting up to 40 perc 30s in a day is over three times the maximum prescribed dose over a 24-

hour period. Taking that many in a day, Sam should be dead a couple times over, but his

tolerance was sky high. Nevertheless, he still had more money than he could spend, so he could

eat as many as he wanted.

With that paranoia came suspicions of police surveillance. By 2011 when he'd been

operating for over a year, government agencies were well-aware of what was happening. They

were beginning to routinely pull over vehicles with out of state plates, putting a bullseye on a 25-

person bus from Ohio. The way around it was simple, once the prescriptions were filled, every

passenger kept their pills on them until arrival back in Ohio. The fear of catching a beating or losing their spot on the bus kept passengers from sneaking any, so pill loss was never an issue, "Everybody kept their own shit and it was kind of like a respect thing, they don't get into it. If you did, then you'd keep an eye on everything. They're not going back next time and they might not get their money or what they want out of it." Even with this plan in place, Sam and his crew were always at risk. There's only so much you can do to insulate yourself when you're violating federal trafficking laws, but he was always cautious, "I'd feel like I was getting heat on me and I'd slow down and I'd go back to [legal] work just to have a routine schedule down and then I can go back [to Florida]." Going back and forth between Florida runs and the cover of a straight job was just about the only thing Sam thought he could do to lay low aside from quitting, and that wasn't going to happen. Eventually, continuing his operation caught up to him,

> What it was is there's a guy that died when I was in Florida and they came to the hotel room, got all of our names and everything else. Then like seven, eight months later, Florida DEA and FBI and all came up to my house [in Ohio], knocking on my door to serve me a subpoena…They tried to tell me that they were going to get me on a federal murder charge because the guy died and I said "How're you going to hit me with a murder charge? I wasn't even in the same room, around him or nothing?"… but I had a pot plant growing outside my house and they hit me with manufacturing drugs for one pot plant because I didn't end up snitching. So, then that's when I went to rehab a couple times. I got convicted for major cultivation and I ended up getting locked. I went to prison for eight months, judicialed out because I was dropping dirty for being on pills, so I was asking for help. I've had three different probation officers and they say, "You keep dropping dirty, we're going to put you in rehab," and I looked at him and I said, "Please do, I want to get off of them." I was doing 40 a day but I got down like two or three 30s a day and I'm like, "I want help." They granted me the workhouse program, but a judge denied me and sent me to prison. That was my first felony, first probation violation and everything, and I was asking for help.

That was back 2013...but they sent me to prison and when I was in there an old charge came back on me where a kid wore wire on me while I was selling pills. So, I judicialed out, got out for four months and they sent me right back for another 18 months. And then ever since I got out then, that was 2015 when I got out there and probably just been getting high, it's like I've just been down, like everything's been against me. It feels like that's what my addictions were telling me like, "Fuck it, you might as well get high. Nothing's going to change." It's like I got stuck in that chain of insanity.

Sam had reached the end of the road. His paranoia turned out to be justified and his operation had landed him on law enforcement's radar, not a surprise given the size and consistency of the runs. The stress was getting to be too much but walking away from that kind of money was difficult. In a sense, the arrest was a sort of inflection point for Sam. By the time he was getting prison terms, he wanted to quit. With each interaction with the system, Sam's cynicism increased, feeling like he wasn't getting the kind of help he needed. Ultimately, counterintuitively, the accumulation of charges pushed him further down the road into addiction.

While Sam was a recent entrant into the world of organized drug sales, pill collection was so lucrative that career drug dealers, with no experience in dealing pills, overhauled their entire business model to capitalize on the fad. Justin (WM31) never got involved in the Florida trips. He'd always sold coke and wanted to keep it that way. It had become a reliable and predictable system, and that was important to him. He'd come from a family of boosters, professional thieves, so he'd learned how to make a quick buck at an early age. He got into the drug game around the time he dropped out of high school at 17 and caught on with an older coke dealer he met through family connections. He showed Justin the ropes and taught him the ins and outs of his business. He was in his late 50s and had been dealing for over 30 years with no arrests, so Justin knew he was for real. Over the next decade, Justin became a fairly prolific dealer, though his luck with the law wasn't quite as good as his mentor's. We'll come back to Justin's story later on, but his connections with other drug sellers meant that he had immediate ties to large Florida operations. While he never got into transportation, Justin eventually became a major wholesale buyer and prolific seller of Florida pills.

> I had a couple buddies tried to get me to do it. I know a lot of people that sell drugs, that that's their career. That's what they've always done. They've never been in trouble, and they basically just go wherever the money's at. Whatever this area is flooded with, that's what they sell.

> I really didn't want to do all the shit that you had to do to get through the hoops. The MRIs. You got to deal with all these fucking people and, I didn't want to deal with all that stuff. I knew they made a lot of money.

> I knew the very first dude that I had started dealing with, that I bought pills from, he had two vans and what he did was a van would go to Florida. It would have 10 people in it. The Ford Econoline, the big vans. He'd send one of those down there. It'd have 10 people in it and that van would get there. Those people would be going to the doctor, another would load up and it would go down, and the first one would come back and they change the oil, plugs, all that shit. Ten more people would get in it and go to Florida. It was just a constant cycle like that– run down and come back. They did that shit for a long time. In the beginning they were getting stupid, ridiculous counts. I mean, they would go down there, each person would get three hundred and some 30s, three hundred and some 15s. I mean, that was each person's count. There'd be eight to ten people in each one of these vans.

> A lot of people that sell drugs never make it anywhere. Once you start moving up and you start buying bigger amounts of weight, you figure, if I buy bricks [of cocaine] from you, I'm not buying one at a time. You know what I mean? … for somebody that is selling, he's actually got bricks, you'd go to his house and you'd get it from him. And for someone to just be like, "You know what, I'm not going to do this no more. I'm going to buy me a couple of vans and I'm just going to fucking

load it up and take people to Florida." I mean, they're making money off of that shit.

The counts were huge. They were paying a dollar or $2 for a perc 30 and the 50 cents or a dollar for a perc 15…No one really knew about it, because I had started getting them before a lot of people knew what 30s were yet.

Then finally I started getting hip to what they're doing. I mean, they're paying a dollar a piece. So, you figure, if he would take someone, just one person, take one person down there and they only got 500 bucks…paid for the room and food, but the script only costs $350…All in all, per person, was like $1,500 for to pay them and to fill the scripts and all that shit. Well, the turn on that was like a $10,000 something or upper $10,000, lower $11,000, something like that.

We buy a brick of coke for $25,000, maybe paying 28– the worst powder. And off of that if you broke it down and sold it in pieces that somebody was going to use, you might make $40,000, but just to buy a brick, if you bought it for 25, it's probably going to sell it for 27. You didn't have none of the overhead of going [to Florida] and all that shit but you figure versus you make $2,000 off of a $25,000 investment and then they turn around and pay $1,500 to make $10,000 off of it.

When that much money is on the line, it's hard to imagine turning down the opportunity– a 600% return on investment in four days. Compared to other forms of contemporaneous drug selling, the discrepancy highlights just how profitable the Florida scheme was. Not to mention, if you get pulled over, a police officer will be less likely to question the legitimacy of a pill prescription. As knowledge of the operation spread, more and more pills hit the street. For a time, the strongest of them remained affordable, resulting in widespread use.

In Ohio, They Were Like Skittles

There was a pill ring, a pill epidemic. A couple of people was going down to Florida and was bringing them back. It was just so plentiful that people were giving them to people. It was like Skittles; you know what I'm saying? *Back then it wasn't even about the money. It was just "I got some of these. You want some of these?"*

- Henry (WM30)

Prescribing statistics in Ohio showed that there had been an uptick in the number of prescriptions written each year after 2006. In that year, there were 87.7 opioid prescriptions written in Ohio per 100 individuals, but that figure peaked at 102.4 in 2010 (CDC 2020). While they showed a meaningful increase, the problem with these statistics is that they weren't an accurate representation of what was really happening. They failed to capture the flood of pills coming into the state that were written and filled in other localities. The majority of users knew about Florida, but many didn't want to get involved. In truth, the sheer volume of what was coming back allowed someone to not participate, yet still reap the rewards.

It didn't take long for people to recognize the scale of what was happening. Anyone with even the weakest of ties to the street heard the buzz connected to Florida. There was likely only a degree of separation between any given pill user and an opioid connection. Ryan (WM49) was one of those people.

> I knew people that sold pills, and that's when people going down to Florida and getting prescriptions and coming up here. When the perc 30s really hit hard in Columbus, I started making friends. I got information of who had pills, where I could get them. So that's when I started buying them on the streets. I had never seen a perc 30 at all until this Florida stuff started. And I had never gone down there, but I was asked. They were getting prescriptions down there, and they could go to a pharmacy and get them. I mean lots and lots of pills and bring them back here and make so much money in Columbus…People were making a lot, a lot of money off that.

Prior to asking his friend, Ryan didn't even know what a Percocet was, let alone what it looked like. It didn't take long for him to get hooked, and when he did, there was no shortage of dealers happy to supply his habit. To him, it seemed like everyone was making the trip down there, so that meant finding someone that was holding was easy, too easy. The more connections he made, the more he learned about the entire operation. While he never made the trip himself, the advancement of his addiction was driven by the sheer volume of pills available to him at low prices.

After she got hooked on pills, Liz (AF34) relied heavily on the supply coming from Florida to sustain her habit too. She had already been getting a consistent script of percs from her doctor, but that wasn't cutting it anymore. She needed much more than she could ever legally get from a single doctor and wasn't keen to start doctor shopping. Luckily, pills weren't hard to find on the street. They weren't even a block away, "I would go to my doctor's appointments every month, get my script. The lady that lived down the corner from of me, she sold them. I'd go in and buy as many as I needed and set off for the day. It was easy. When the opioid flood hit Ohio, it was everywhere…All my friends were doing it, so they had pills. The people I mostly went to, they always had them." With such easy access, she could buy as many as percs as she could afford. Socially, when everyone that she knew was on them, it seemed normal enough to be taking them, even at the rate that she escalated to (Kelly et al. 2017). There were times where she questioned what she was doing, but quickly dismissed any reservations. In her mind, she wasn't doing anything wrong; the percs she bought came from people she knew well before her addiction began and the pills were the same as what she got from her doctor, which made it feel normal.

Kelly (WF27) had a somewhat similar experience in the development of her pill use. Through a combination of implicit normativity and sheer abundance of Florida percs, her habit swiftly escalated before she fully understood what she was doing.

> I know part of it was because I had unlimited access to them. My dad had hundreds of them, and he would leave, go out of town with his girlfriend [on pill runs], and leave me there to sell them to his people. And I'm like, "Well, if I wanted one, I could just go get one." They were just there…more than I could ever do anything with. There were so many of them. Just bottles and bottles and bottles of them. Back then, they were cheap. Dirt cheap. I mean, a 30 milligram Percocet was $12. They're $40 now. I don't know how anybody could afford to do them now. They're so expensive. But I had them, they were literally at my fingertips, hundreds of them.

At such a young age, the temptation to try the percs was too much of a draw for Kelly to resist. There was clearly a reason why her family kept bringing them back from Florida and why they sold out as quickly as they did upon return. With so many pills on hand, she knew her dad would never know if she snuck a few here and there. The problem was that it didn't stop there, and she developed a raging addiction before she had fully come to terms with what she was on and how much her body craved them. When she did, there was a problem. Dad stopped bringing them back from Florida. He wasn't the only one. Progressively, vans that used be on the road consistently were parked, empty. Doctor's offices were getting hit by law enforcement, slowly taking the go-to clinics off the board (Kennedy-Hendricks et al. 2015). As she mentioned, stable demand without the expected supply created a spike in prices, drastically impacting addicts that depended on the market.

All good things must come to an end. For illicit pill users in Ohio, that time was the mid-2010s. Regulation and enforcement efforts initiated in the years prior started the ball rolling, but there was a substantial burden to overcome before changes sent a meaningful ripple through drug markets. Law enforcement was stepping up opioid-focused interventions, and users were taking notice. Contemporaneously, at the policy level, doctors faced pressure to overhaul prescribing behaviors. Faced with the newly-dubbed "Opioid Epidemic," change was essential (Smith 2017; Weisberg et al. 2014). While true, it's likely an overcorrection took place. It's no coincidence that there was an exponential increase in the number of overdose deaths corresponding with a linear decrease in the number of scripts being written (Jalal et al. 2018). Individuals that had received the pills for years developed dependencies, especially among those that used the pills beyond the prescribed amount (i.e., just about everyone in my sample that got pills from a doctor). In combination with one another, both legal and regulatory pressures changed the landscape of opioid use. Without pharmaceutically dispensed supply, users were forced to turn to the streets, introducing variability and risk regarding what they were getting that had not existed previously. Street prices of pills soared, and users were getting sick more often. Even if they had the cash, tracking the pills down was becoming more and more difficult. As a result of the worsening drought and widespread elimination or reduction of personal scripts, many found themselves on a fast track to heroin.

Max's (WM34) situation was a quintessential example of how the abrupt elimination of an opioid prescription could have life-altering effects. Before his addiction, Max had been a successful business owner with over a hundred employees, but a car crash changed all of that. He barely survived the accident, and he came away with the injuries to prove it, "I had multiple fractures in my face. Broke my left collar bone in five places. Three broken ribs. Collapsed lung. Collapsed stomach. Left wrist was broke. Left forearm was broke. Fractures in my knees. It took me two months. I was two months in the hospital learning how to walk and talk again." Throughout his hospitalization, Max had been administered large doses of opioids intravenously, since the injuries to his face and jaw made taking pills impossible. Once he was able, he was shifted onto perc 30s through the time he was discharged.

Max's real problems started when the doctors decided he didn't need the pills anymore. After two years on the percs, he had become highly dependent. He still had constant pain and found himself trying to outrun his increasing tolerance. The pressure of trying to save a failing business caused him to use well beyond his prescribed daily dosage, up to the point where what he was taking enough to kill the average non-user. There was no warning, just a notice that the pharmacy was not authorized to fill his prescription, and he felt betrayed.

> It was pretty much the doctors. They would tell you the laws are getting stricter, "We're not allowed to prescribe this many anymore." "I'm going to have to lower your dosage." "We're no longer doing long-term treatments." "They're not made for long-term anymore." It was just more or less why? Okay, you guys put me on these. You know the type of injuries I have. The injuries say that they're never going to go away or get better. You guys are telling me I'm going to be in pain for the rest of my life, but you want me to cut back on medication because the laws are stricter now? So how is that beneficial to me?

Max was upset, and he had the right to be– to an extent. While he never had a choice regarding whether he was started on the pills, he was never told to take his pills at such an accelerated rate either. His unmonitored self-medicating had left him in an incredibly vulnerable position where he needed a considerable number to stay well, all of which now had to come from the street.

In the months after, his life rapidly deteriorated. Predictably, Max wasn't able to get his hands on enough pills each day. He was sick all the time. Sweating, shaking, vomiting, diarrhea–there was no more ignoring Max's situation. He was a drug addict and everyone around him knew it.

> I lost everything. I had my kids taken away. I was pretty much on pain pills, couldn't afford them, was doing limited amounts, was in extreme pain, got introduced to heroin, it was cheap. I was hearing everybody say how bad it was. It was like, "I'll never go to that. I'll never go to that. I don't care if I spend every dollar on pain pills." Then eventually, I just couldn't take it. They were too hard to get anymore. If you did get them, they were fake. People were re-pressing them. So, it was like, "Well, I'm just going to snort heroin instead of injecting it." Then it went from that to injecting.

Max was on prescription pills for an extended period, abused them, was taken off the pills, bought them off the street until he couldn't find and/or afford them, and switched to heroin. He didn't want to, but he didn't feel like he had much of a choice either.

Others experienced a similar pathway, ultimately culminating with IV heroin use. Sean (WM36) suffered from a degenerative joint condition that had caused him pain for as long as he could remember. Percs were the only thing that kept the pain somewhat in check, but even those had their limitations. Over the years, his tolerance increased, as did his dosage. Then, suddenly, his prescription was terminated. He wasn't buying them off the street yet, largely because he was on a sizeable daily intake and had some to spare. However, changing regulations deemed that ibuprofen was sufficient, leaving Sean scrambling for pills.

> Restrictions were harder. It wasn't like I could just go down the street now and find Dr. Bob and he'll just continue giving me Oxycodone 30s. My doctor's probably going to be like, "What the fuck are you doing on these? You got

cancer?" So, I couldn't find another doctor, so I'm suddenly sick. I was looking for other doctors, but they either weren't taking patients, or the state was shutting them down. The vendors, some of the south end pill mills, they were shutting them down. I got some through my network of people that I knew were getting pain pills, but all of a sudden, doctors were being restricted that they can only have a certain percentage of patients on pain pills. If not, by this time you had to go to a pain clinic. You think about that as a dope addict– we can't even hardly be on time for anything. Trying to go through all these appointments just to maybe get pills, it was easier for me to go to the street and buy them…but the supply was dwindling. 2015 is when prices of Percocets, pain pills, was going up. Supply was definitely going down, and I'd lost my own supply. And then my friend on the west side, he's like, "Well, come out. I got you." I was sick, so I drive to his house. This is January of 2015. I'm like, "What have you got? I'll buy some." He's like, "Oh, I don't got pain pills, but I got pure opiates." And he pulls it out. This is this is the first time I've ever seen heroin in my life. First time ever…Next thing I know, I'm sitting in the kitchen getting my arm tied up. She's doing it, and that first shot…I mean, the next day I overdosed in his house. It escalated quick. All of a sudden, I'm an IV user of heroin, and never looked back.

While he still had his script, Sean had things under some semblance of control; he was addicted, but his supply from a legitimate source kept him on the straight and narrow. Once that source was removed, everything changed. Desperation took over. Sean wasn't alone either. He saw the same thing happening to everyone else, it seemed. For a short time, he could get pills from the street, but those ran out as well. He relentlessly searched for them, only to arrive at a constrained choice: enduring the sickness or using heroin.

Amy (WF31) eventually found herself using heroin as well. Her wholesale pill connections kept getting hit by the police, throwing a wrench into a well-oiled system that had made her quite a bit of money middlemanning for friends and acquaintances. Of course, she got hooked on the percs along the way and had an advanced habit by the time she noticed

enforcement was ramping up. She burned her bridges to medical sources years prior, but still

relied on a flawed system to generate the product her supplier provided her. When that was no

longer viable, she stopped selling. Amy had money back then, but it got to a point where that

didn't even matter. There was nothing to spend it on.

> It was hard to get pills. Police were cracking down… it was like something just
> happened. People were having trouble getting them. Then people were selling
> fake ones that were like laundry soap and just dyeing them. And we had lost a
> whole bunch of money. Then, I was very adamant on never doing heroin. And I'll
> never forget the first time that I did it was I came home from work and I was sick.
> And my boyfriend was sitting at the coffee table and he told me that it was
> chopped up Percocet. That it was already grinded down. It was white. Percs are
> blue. I knew. But in my mind, I didn't want to know. I was sick and I didn't care.
> It just kind of escalated from there. Once you do it the first time, you feel so good,
> you're like, "Does it even matter? It's cheaper. This is way more accessible. Pills
> are impossible to get now. Doctors are cracking down. Nobody's giving them out
> anymore."

The combination of enforcement attention and the changing regulation of doctors shook Amy's

world. Her source of income was gone, as was her usual source. Without the percs, she turned to

the street. She had connections from having been involved in selling for a few years, but

everyone was finding themselves in a similar position. They, like Amy, had needs, both personal

and professional, and nowhere to turn but heroin.

Mason (WM32) got hooked on percs as a result of recreational experimentation. He only

ever received a script long after he became addicted. Over the first couple years of his addiction,

his pill habit escalated to over $300 per day, and that was before the spike. In the course of a few

weeks, pills became harder to find and prices were quickly rising. Just about everyone he knew in his neighborhood was on pills, meaning that competition for whatever was available was stiff. Word started to spread about what was happening in Florida, that law enforcement was shutting down many of the clinics that Ohio operators had become dependent upon,

> Everybody was aware of the DEA because they let it be known. You'd go out to Florida and go to your doctor and your doctor's like, "Well, DEA's cracking down." So then word just spreads. And then you notice the pills ain't so plentiful as they was. It just got a lot of people hooked on heroin. It's definitely their fault, the reason why the heroin epidemic took off like it did. Because what they did...I mean its peoples' fault for doing it, doing the pills, and then switching over…But they [companies] made it. They contributed to the heroin epidemic because they made it so easy for everybody to get pills. They just let them go long enough to get you hooked on them, and then they just pulled them right back. And then "Boom." That's when heroin took off...Because I grew up here. I heard about heroin every once in a while. I never in my life seen heroin. And then all of the sudden, the pill shit started going on. And you know, then once that happened, that's when I actually started seeing the heroin everywhere. Because I grew up in the hood and I never seen heroin my whole life until after that pill shit happened.

Reflecting on his trajectory after the fact, Mason retraced how things fell apart for him. It all started with the pills. When they were plentiful, life was great. When they were scarce, not so much. He took a turn for the worse. He wasn't thinking clearly. His unsatisfied addiction prohibited it. He needed a fix and heroin was the answer, the only answer. He couldn't help but be bitter about it. After several felonies and a family destroyed, his life was forever changed. What started as having a good time ended with rampant heroin use. As he said, that was all new. Prior to the pill shortage, heroin was never on anyone's mind. He would have known. He lived in one of the worst neighborhoods in the city and drug selling was ubiquitous. But when the faucet was turned off, he, as well as most of his friends and family, were all desperate to stay well.

Chapter 2. Graduation: I Never Thought I'd Do Heroin

"I only knew a couple of people that went straight to heroin. But most of the people I know went through that phase where it was getting painkillers first, then getting cut off their painkillers, then buying painkillers on the streets, and it was really expensive, then they just switched to heroin. So, it was like a little transition, not just jumping straight to heroin."

- Josh (WM26)

Arriving at heroin was most often the end result of several stages of opioid use, heavily influenced by external factors. It was a progression. When pills began to dry up and addicts couldn't afford what they could find, they were likely to start using heroin. It was cheaper, more effective, and most importantly, it was available. There was a catch. The stigma associated with heroin use was immense. It's the point of no return. There's no more pretending that you're just "having a good time" or you've got everything "under control." Pills, on the other hand, were safe. Acceptable even. Moving beyond them required a reframing of a one's self-image, a reckoning that many addicts try to outrun. Letting go of the idea of who you used to be was an unsettling process, but it's one that every graduating pill user endured sooner or later.

From the Doctor: The Legitimacy of Pills and the Facilitation of Addiction

The doctor wrote it for me, so it's got to be okay. It's got to be what I need. They went to college, I didn't. They graduated high school. I just got a GED. They know a lot more than me. I was ignorant like that, for real.

- Sam (WM41)

The vast majority of individuals that take painkillers do so responsibly and never develop a dependency or addiction. However, for individuals predisposed to addiction-related disorders, exposure carries a higher likelihood of addiction (Hasin et al. 2013; O'Brien 2003). Deficient impulse control becomes especially problematic when it exists within the context that engenders legitimacy. Individuals like Sam, who went on to operate a prolific Florida pill mill scheme, put trust in his doctors that we as a society are conditioned to afford them. It's expected, and for good reason. Someone that has gone to medical school carries the sort of knowledge of anatomy that makes them uniquely qualified for their profession. But, as in all things human, what happens when they make a mistake?

For so many pill users, that mistake meant exposure to a prescription that would ultimately lead them to a horribly destructive chemical dependency. Much of the burden of responsible use is certainly on the patient, but for many in my sample, the subject of addiction never came up with doctors. No warning that the pills have the potential to be addictive, no consideration of any prior periods of addiction, and no discussion of how the pills share properties with heroin. That last part is especially problematic. The word "heroin" carries a great deal of stigma. Any mention of that word snaps a patient to attention.

Because pills are legally manufactured and require a prescription, it gives them the sort of legitimacy that few other addictive substances can equal. Because they're medicine used to treat ailments, they have credibility among individuals that would otherwise view drug use as being incompatible with their belief structure. Using painkillers is socially acceptable. Pills played a large role in Adam's downfall. He didn't realize that pills caused sickness the same way that heroin would until it was too late. After that, he was never the same again. But the pills had come from the doctor, so they weren't really a drug. How bad could something be if a doctor gives it to you? That mentality was a slippery slope. For some, they saw the pills just like any other bottle of pills– if your head still hurts, just take another Tylenol. Applying the same thinking to opioids is a recipe for disaster, but it didn't stop it from happening. As a person's tolerance went up, it became increasingly common for people like Todd (WM36) to look to additional pills to help dull pain,

> I got my tolerance built up and I was still getting breakthrough pain. So, I'd take another one, and take another one. It got to the point where the hours didn't matter to me, it was when I got in pain, that's when I'm taking another one. If I was away and I didn't have them with me or whatever and I was in pain, I'd get home, I eat one and then I'd snort one. That way it would kick in fast and take the pain away.

Even when they moved beyond eating them to snorting them, addicts like Todd still framed their drug abuse as treatment for pain (Daniulaityte et al. 2012). It didn't matter that what he was doing wasn't on the side of the bottle, it was what worked. Because it was a prescription, Todd allowed his "addict brain" to minimize what was happening. He had become a drug addict, but to him, he just required more medicine.

Todd wasn't alone in adopting a warped interpretation of pill consumption that kept their use going. Steve (WM44) had been on the pills for several months before things started to come apart. He'd been using them following a lengthy hospital stay for a work-related accident. As he recuperated, he started to question whether he still truly needed the pills.

> I needed it. My body needed that shit. That's what I thought in my mind. Really, that's what I thought. Honestly, it didn't…I definitely would've got healed faster if I wasn't on all that medicine. I thought I was in pain. I had to take these. "The doctor gives me these. These are from the doctor." That's how I justified them in my head…But I don't need them now. I don't need nothing. I'm not even taking Aspirin, you know what I mean?

Steve had standing refills for three pain doctors'-worth of prescriptions, so supply wasn't a problem. He knew and ignored the reality of his situation, but he justified his use as faithful adherence to the treatment plan given to him by his doctors– even though the fact that he had multiple doctors was problematic in and of itself. He didn't need the pills anymore, but, whether conscious or not, he knew that he didn't need to stop either. He still had several months' supply with his name on it, that was, until he didn't.

Tamika (BF29) found herself in a similar situation. She ruptured her appendix, requiring surgery and a considerable amount of recuperation. During her recovery, she popped several of her stitches and, while she'll admit it wasn't all that bad, it was enough to get her a second script from her doctor's assistant. Within a few weeks, Tamika had healed completely, but she still had a considerable number of refills left. Like Steve, she was at a point where she felt fine. Even still, she wasn't quite ready to stop the pills and, just to be safe, she figured that she should listen to her doctor and keep taking them, "I just felt the doctor knew. Like, okay, you need to take them for a certain period of time. So, I never really thought about it. I did not even know they would be considered a drug until later on but just something so you will not be in pain. I thought everybody got it." Even though she was in no pain, she was able to justify using them by attributing her lack of pain to the pills. By creating her own version of the chicken-and-egg, she could continue taking the pills guilt-free.

For Dirty People: The Stigma of Heroin and the Intensity of Resistance

> *I was trying to justify– I'm doing pills. At least it ain't heroin. I'm better than heroin. I was spending 10 times more for sure. Pills are so much more expensive than heroin. A perc 10 can go for $18 apiece, and I would buy 10, sometimes 20 of them a day. You know what I mean? If I spend $100 on some heroin, that can last me a couple days. I would buy 10, 20 pills, and that would only last me one day. The stigma was big. Really*

was. Because I knew what it was going to lead to…my sister was on it really bad, and I seen what her life was becoming.

- Josh (WM26)

Nothing underscores the perceived legitimacy of pills like heroin. Chemically, they're not so different. In practice, enough pills can at least approximate a heroin high. Mentally, however, they could not be more dissimilar. Josh eventually graduated to heroin. He resisted it for as long as he could, but at a certain point, he had to give in. He fought tooth and nail. He backed it up with his wallet. He was willing to pay *ten times more* for pills rather than be perceived as someone that uses dope. He knew that he could have a stronger drug for a fraction of the price, but it was unthinkable. Being addicted to pills was bad but being addicted to heroin was something else entirely. It was the lowest of the low. Even hardcore pill addicts like Josh looked down on heroin use. They knew that heroin was going to be the beginning of a downward spiral that was likely to destroy their lives– they'd seen it happen before. Family members, people from your neighborhood, hookers standing on the corner, you couldn't miss it. In spite of firsthand knowledge of what was awaiting them, they took the plunge.

The ability to disassociate from deviant behavior by contrasting it against even worse deviant behavior is a curious proposition. It represents another step further away from normalcy, whether it's admitted to or not. During pill use, denial was still viable, but it was hard to not recognize what was transpiring. They were running through prescriptions faster and their tolerances were climbing, both of which are perceptible changes. It's not like misplacing your car keys. Even then, the justification for nearly everyone, including Joel (WM35), was that the pills weren't actually all that bad because they weren't heroin– drug addicts use heroin.

Pain pills it felt, or I imagined it like a white-collar drug, everybody's doing it, doctors, lawyers, whoever. And heroin, I always pictured it being people laying in the street and shooting up in alleys and overdosing or whatever. I don't know, it just seemed *dirty*. Seeing people on heroin around my neighborhood, seeing what they looked like. I was doing good when I first did the pain pills. Still in my head at the time I was feeling like the pain pills were helping me, and it didn't feel like it was hurting.

Everyone was doing pills; good people were doing pills. If you still had your shit together, even in the smallest sense, you were still able to take solace in knowing that you weren't one of *them*. They're doing heroin. They're bad people. For Joel, this was an important exercise in cognitive dissonance. Since he started using 15 years prior, he'd had an estimated 25 drug arrests, hardly leaving his status as a law-abiding citizen in question. But in his mind, he wasn't on heroin, so how bad could he really be?

The internal distinction between good and bad was pervasive. Pill use existed as a mechanism to reinforce that boundary. Joseph (WM30) felt similarly to Joel, believing that the legality of pills was something that differentiated his behavior from street drug users, in spite of all of his pills coming from the street,

I think it's just associated with heroin being *dirty*, needles, all that. The thing about pills, pills come from the manufacturer. They're government marketed...I mean, so it gets down to that. And once you start using heroin, you use it so much, you're considered a dope fiend. Once you pretty much associate with something like that, you're just labeled as a *dirty* person, a heroin addict. You know what I mean? Why would I want to be labeled like that? I'm too good for that type of thing…it goes hand-in-hand with just trash. It's just, you don't want to be labeled like that. You don't want to feel that way.

Once you start to use heroin, your perception in the eyes of others changes. In communities that have consistent exposure to what a dope fiend looks like, the last thing you want is to be funneled into that same category by your peers. In that sense, paying ten times as much for an inferior product comes into clarity. It's not just about the high. More importantly, it's all of the baggage that's attached to one, but not the other. Do pills, maintain your status. Do heroin, lose it all.

The need to distance oneself from heroin use was something that had to be expressed openly, to be modeled in front of others in order to reinforce which side of the boundary you stood on. Even the slightest suggestion that you were a heroin user in a public space necessitated a strong rebuke, dare one look indifferent to the distinction. One day, while hanging out with her friends, Raquel (BF42) had this sort of situation arise, "I remember somebody actually offering me some heroin. I was like, 'What the fuck is that?' When they told me, I went, 'Fuck off!' That's how much like of a stigma. It was just, 'How dare you disrespect me like that?' Fuck. Horrible. Like, 'How dare you? You know who I am?'"

On a private level, Raquel had a somewhat negative view of heroin. But in public? She had to "shut that shit down;" leave no doubt in anyone's mind how she felt about the drug. Even though she'd been a consistent drug user since age 14, had a well-developed pill and methadone addiction, and had sold most of her life, all of that was on a different, lower level. She hadn't yet graduated to heroin. It would only be a few months after this confrontation until she made the transition. She'd thought about it for years, but resisting it was integral to her sense of where she belonged and the maintenance of her reputation.

Kathy (WF44) had never been in trouble before, making the maintenance of her image as "normal" person essential. When her pill use started, she lived with an abusive husband and her two kids in a double-wide in North Carolina. They weren't well off, but she thought they had a life that was more-or-less okay. She started hearing about the pain pills coming out of Florida and how they were becoming more popular throughout Appalachia. She'd already been getting them from a friend and taking them recreationally for a few months, not really fully understanding what she was on.

> It was a massive problem in North Carolina down to Florida at that time in the United States. Yeah, I read up on it. It's where it started, I think with the pill mills down in Florida and then all the way up. They were legal so when people call it hillbilly heroin, I was like, "I'd never do heroin. These are legal. I'm a good drug addict with kids." You know what I mean? So, the stigma, it just wasn't there [with pills]. I would never have touched heroin back then. The pills were legal and they were like, appropriate. Heroin addicts shoot up. I could take a pill like a normal person, like a lady, and I could drive, care for children, go to college, work, live my best life whereas a junkie was in an alley on the ground with the needle in his arm dying. And I certainly was not that person. Even when I was a housewife, it was okay to take pills because I was bored. I would take one. My friend would take one. We'd get our toddlers together and we would enrich these children's lives by reading to them and letting them play in the pool while we were high as fuck. We'd just pop a pill and go on about painting our fingernails. So, we acted appropriately.

The first thing that her investigation into pills yielded was that they were becoming a problem and that one half of a common moniker was "heroin." Even still, it was fine. Her habit was different. There's a long history of the "bored housewife on pills" trope dating back to the 50s and the social acceptability of prescription use. To Kathy, this was just a modern extension. People can call it hillbilly heroin if they want, but that's just their opinion. She knew she wasn't doing *actual* heroin. These were legal and came from a doctor, even though hers did not, but they could have. She was still able to maintain her family, pursue her education, and care for her kids.

There was nothing inappropriate in that, she thought. But, just like Raquel, she ended up

shooting heroin.

In the eyes of other parents, using the pills was a socially acceptable activity to engage in.

Moving beyond pills, however, wasn't something that was acceptable for a parent. We learned a

bit about Keisha's (MF38) backstory earlier, that her absentee mother, in more ways than one,

contributed to her drug use as a teenager. After getting clean and having a kid, a series of five

auto accidents in one year had her back on pills, but her treatment did her more harm than good.

Unfortunately, her reintroduction to the pills spurred a period of opioid addiction that lasted from

2003 to 2019, 16 years, and drastically altered her trajectory. It wasn't long until she progressed

to heroin, but even then, she desperately tried to conceal her use, knowing what it could mean if

word got around. She was less concerned with status at this point, but instead with what a

"heroin user" label might mean as a parent,

> I thought that if people still just thought I did pills they wouldn't judge me. If I'm
> on heroin, because I've got my kids and stuff…people overdosing, or the stuff
> people say. When I thought heroin, I thought needles. It just seemed like people
> would frown upon you more for heroin than pills. But it's kind of the same thing,
> opioid-wise. I'm still maintaining. I was still going to work. On the outside, I was
> still taking care of what I had to do. But as soon as they would have heard I was
> on heroin they would be like, "Oh no." You know what I mean? People will start
> looking at you a different way. Start calling Children Services on you or whatever
> they do. Because heroin was always that, "Oh, that drug is worse than that drug.
> That drug is worse." And it always was heroin. Supposedly the worst drug of all
> time. I couldn't just pull out the heroin, right? Start shooting in front of people.

Kathy was a mom on pills, but she was able to hide behind the prescription label. Having

graduated to heroin, Keisha knew she was no longer protected by benefit of the doubt. She was aware of the ramifications that accompany the stigma of a parent on heroin and how important it was to keep it a secret because of how damaging it could be. Get caught, they take the kids. Every time.

Internal Bargaining and Moving the Line

> *Kevin (WM23): We went on a Percocet kick that lasted for maybe a month and a half, doing a couple a day. Then we couldn't find any…There's a lot of rightfully placed stigma around heroin. It started two-, two-and-a-half years of absolute misery. After it started, I don't know if I thought about it too much, the stigma. I justified it just like, "Well that'll never be me. I'm only using it this much. Snorting it versus shooting. I'm only doing this or that, so there's no way I could ever end up like that person. Right? I'm not going to end up as desperate or destitute as so and so." It was like arbitrary lines drawn in the sand that all got crossed later on. But that was justification for me feeling like, "Well, everything's under control right now. We still have the apartment, and we still have these material things." Just rationalization for behavior that I'm sure I knew was wrong. I mean, internally, there are multiple times where I was like, "This is untenable. I want to be done with this because what we're doing isn't sustainable and somebody's going to die or we're going to end up in prison." I just couldn't stop.*

> *Q: When those lines in the sand got crossed or moved, was that something that you thought about, or did it affect you in any way?*

> *Kevin: Nope. Not at all. Honestly, it's just when it got crossed, it was just almost exciting. Your body knows. Any time I cross a line, especially towards the end, I didn't need to rationalize anything for myself. It was more so just like, "This is what it is, and this is what it has to be." Because I don't want to be sick and I don't know any other way. Really, like the rationalization and stuff was at the beginning when I'm still trying to justify my behavior. And I'm like, "Well, it's just like pills. It's just the wrong form." You know what I mean?" Stupid logics like that.*

The concept of "the line" was pervasive, existing as a series of empty promises to oneself. Crossing the line in an absolute, binary sense meant defeat. Kicking the can down the road meant not having to face that reality. For example, altering "I'm only on pills, I'll never use heroin" to "I might be snorting heroin, but I'll never shoot it," a person can maintain a connection to who they wish they still were, something that Kevin tried to do. Ultimately, like so many, he failed.

The advancement of opioid abuse is a bargaining exercise. A series of successive deals, each one becoming increasingly tenuous. For people like Kevin, a line in the sand was flexible to the point of meaninglessness. Any given line just ended up being a suggestion. You feel guilty for not complying, but you disregard it all the same. Nearly everyone made the transition to heroin use, largely attributable to a lack of pills, and wrestling with that reality made many feel like a piece of shit for it, a sentiment Amy (WF31) expressed.

> I just felt like that [shooting] was for *dirty* people. It was for junkies and I wasn't a junkie. I just felt like if I put a needle in my arm, then that was the line. I think I've always drawn lines. Like, "If I don't do this, then I'm not a bad person." You know what I mean? And then when I jumped that line, it's like, "Well, if I don't do this, then I'm not a bad person." It's just kind of like that fake line that makes you feel like you're not a shit bag. That you're in control. *It always moved.* There was always something else that I could be. Like, "Well, at least I'm not doing that." I'd always just find a different set of people to say that I was better than to make myself feel better.

The stigma of heroin was enormous. It kept Amy on pills for over five years. After graduating, the line needed to move. The pressure of perceiving herself as a bad person on the wrong side of the line demanded it. It was too uncomfortable. It wasn't about heroin– it had to become not shooting heroin. It was denial, but it served its purpose. She felt like she was in control again, even if it was a fleeting notion.

Previously, we saw how Steve (WM44) maintained his pill habit out of a naïve, semi-conscious adherence to his prescription pill regimen. They were from his doctor, so it was okay to keep taking them even after he didn't need them. Eventually, he had to face that he had become truly addicted to the pills after three years on them.

> It took about three years just using medicine, like pain medicine and stuff like that before I actually got on heroin. And then it took like two years before I started shooting. I always promised myself, I would never shoot dope, you know what I mean? I'd never do that. Never do that. After you snort for so long, you don't feel that shit the same. Never. I wanted a different high…I felt like I was a piece of shit. That's how I felt about it. Typical drug addict.

Switching to heroin was something he didn't want, but he got there all the same. Now that he was snorting it, he moved the line, now demarcating the boundary between himself and injecting it. He would *never* do it, he thought. But after a while, snorting it wasn't working either. The curiosity of what shooting might be like crept in and bested his resolve. Just like that, he'd broken every promise he'd made to himself and he felt the weight of that realization.

It Just Made Sense: Making the Switch and a Warped Sense of Practicality

> *When the Florida connection got stopped, people were really getting hammered down on prescribing pills. Yeah, it was about '13, '14, about six, seven years ago. So, there was a really dry spell on the streets. I couldn't find any kind of pills anywhere. I was sick, real sick. Went through the withdrawals, went through all that hell, and got to a point where I wasn't sick. I still had all these problems with the relationship and everything, so I needed something to escape from it...I called my guy one day and asked him if he had any*

pills, he said "no." But he said he had some– I'd always told myself I would never go to heroin. I knew addicts– and he said he had some heroin. Probably pretty much without even thinking I said, "Well, I'll get a little bit." And I bought $20 worth and snorted a little bit of it, and I like it. It lasted me all day, and I was thinking, "$20 and it lasts me all day, and I'm spending hundreds a day on pills." I started thinking, "Why didn't I do this sooner?" And it took off from there.

- Ryan (WM49)

The answer to Ryan's question was that his life imploded not long after he started using heroin, but he wasn't alone in asking it. Like the others, Ryan's vehement opposition to graduating to heroin could only last so long. Pill users in my sample often reached a breaking point where "I would never" was set aside. External pressures, pitted against worsening withdrawal symptoms, played a substantial role in that decision. Switching wasn't a spontaneous internal failure. It was typically some combination of an inability to find pills, their prohibitive price, the affordability of heroin, or all of the above. Ryan's experience was common. Users that had previously relied on the flood of out-of-state pills endured a shock when the supply dried up. Making matters worse, around the same time, in-state doctors were tightening pill restrictions as well, further increasing the deficit they needed to cover in order to stay well.

Perhaps the highest hurdle for addicts was finding anyone that had pills. It didn't take long for it to get so dire that it felt as if they had disappeared entirely. On the street, percs were effectively extinct. Sick and seeing no alternatives, pill addicts like Jennifer (WF31) gave in when her back was against the wall, "The first time I did it, and I will never forget it, I remember I couldn't find a pill. I called everybody. I was running around from house to house out West looking for it. Couldn't find it. I did a line of dope with some guy and then probably three days after I snorted it, 'Oh, I'll never shoot it. I'll never shoot it.' Three days later I shot it." Jennifer never wanted to graduate to heroin, but she was sick. She'd been doing pills for a few years, so she had well-developed connections on her side of town, making exhausting possible leads a meaningful action. She tried to avoid dope, but she did what she felt she had to do. Ending her sickness came at a cost though, landing her several felony charges over the next year.

She wasn't alone. Users knew that supply was going down. Either you can't find any or you notice that what 30s you do find, that used to go for $15-20, were now anywhere from $30-40. For a veteran user like Ron (WM37), who regularly spent $300 a day on pills, that was problematic. He'd owned a flourishing carpentry business before he got hooked when he started doing them with his sister, but the increasing cost of his habit necessitated the sale of all of his equipment, including four relatively new Ford trucks. He'd only gotten a fraction of their worth and what money he did receive got crushed up and went straight up his nose. Money was tight and he was out of assets, making heroin an appealing alternative, "By then, the pills are, they're cracking down on the pills. Pills are getting hard to find, they're way more expensive now. It's like, 'Why are you gonna buy pills when you can just buy this? Save yourself some money and have the same thing, if not better.' I'm thinking, I'm the smart one. 'You're an idiot for buying these pills, man. I'm buying dope, saving some money.' You know?" Heroin wasn't just a good deal; it was the *smart* thing to do. In the midst of addiction, this sort of logic seems foolproof to someone in Ron's shoes. Predictably, after a series of arrests, he eventually realized that his assessment of the situation wasn't entirely accurate. Even still, at the time, his options were extremely limited. He was broke, sick, and couldn't find enough pills to satisfy his cravings even if he wanted to.

Embracing the value of heroin in spite of the stigma it carried was much easier with a friend to shepherd you into it. Earl (BM33) grew up in a family of drug dealers and followed in their footsteps, taking over the family business. He became consumed with the lifestyle– cars, jewelry, clothes, and especially how they seemed to attract beautiful women. Especially concerned with material things, he was always open to saving money where he could. When he first heard of heroin, he responded negatively, as most do, but having a close friend on it left him curious.

> I still was doing percs and he was just like, "Hey, man, I've got this heroin." I'm like, "Nuh-uh. I don't want to"… But I did it. It tasted weird and I'm like, "Damn, it got the same buzz and I barely hit this shit." That's how I graduated, because I was introduced by another user that graduated, that used to be on percs with me. He was like, "Fuck that. Ain't make no sense for me paying 60 bucks when I can get a $10 bag and be just as high as you." *All that made sense*, so it was all about the income. It was all about the money. I knew him. I knew him since just a child, childhood friend. If you're doing it every day, it's going to graduate. You're going to gradually go up…if I still had the money to buy Percocet, I'd buy Percocet. But since it continued to be $30, $40 for a perc 30 when I'm going out and get two grams of heroin for it. I did that.

It was a no-brainer. A few years of using percs created a riches-to-rags situation for Earl, so cost-cutting was a must. After he'd overcome the stigma, largely facilitated by a personal introduction, and experienced comparable effects heroin provided, he was sold. Even though he would have preferred to remain on the Percocet, the monetary advantage that heroin provided won out.

For some pill users, the stress of trying to locate 30s and then having to pay for them as well became too much. Simply put, it became too much of a pain in the ass. Guys like Jacob (WM39) got fed up with having to chase them down, often times just to feel somewhat less sick. He had better options,

I was doing a lot of pills. So, the cost was astronomical. Heroin's cheaper. It's still prepared the same way, I'm going to crush it down, I'm going to snort a line of it or whatever. It wasn't like my technique had changed. I knew they were both opioids. I knew one was pharmaceutically made and the other was man made or processed. It just wasn't this big jump for me. Even though the name of it was…that was a scary moment for me, as far as moving into it. But it was so much cheaper and because the war on drugs had ramped up- they started cutting down [on pills]. Pills were harder to get. They started making different forms of them to where you couldn't crush and snort. So, there was this change in the dynamics with pills. And that seemed riskier than getting heroin because the cops are really on pills and…I could get heroin anywhere. I knew I could just talk to the boy on the street and get that. Versus pills, I'd have to know somebody whose great aunt had cancer or something, and I'd have to go through her. You've got to jump through some hoops for sure.

Heroin became the path of least resistance. The first time was scary, but just like Earl, after that it became business as usual for Jacob. It had been unshrouded. Rather than having to go through the process of locating an obscure medical source for pills, he could go to any number of corners and get exactly what he wanted. On top of that, increased legal intervention targeting pills made buying heroin feel safer, carrying a lesser risk of getting caught.

PART II. Can Punishment Work?

Chapter 3. Deterring Crime

Deterrence principles have permeated modern criminal justice policy over the past half century. Through the 1970s, support for rehabilitative corrections eroded as politicians and a new generation of criminologists engaged in increasingly critical examinations of policies that had sought to address socially-rooted contributors to criminality (American Friends Service Committee 1971; Hirsch 1976). In its place, many came to embrace a model based upon deterrence and incapacitation, exemplified by mandatory sentencing, harsher sentencing, and an emphasis on proactive policing (Garland 2001). As a result, such practices substantially increased the number of persons with criminal records (Petersilia 2003) and directly contributed to the growth of mass incarceration (Gottschalk 2006, 2016). Further, much of this growth in prison populations has been attributed to the development and enforcement of draconian drug policy, packaged as a "War on Drugs" (Alexander 2012; Garland 2001; Gottschalk 2016).

At present, the War continues. As of 2018, 32 percent of all incarcerated offenders were incarcerated on drug charges (452,900 inmates). In fact, more individuals are currently incarcerated on drug charges than were incarcerated for all crimes in 1980 (The Sentencing Project 2018). At its core, the underlying premise of deterrence is simple: a would-be offender can be dissuaded from committing a crime if the perceived risk of arrest and the ensuing punishment outweighs the subjective value of a potential reward (Becker 1968). Despite having many critics (Bowling 1999; De Haan and Vos 2003; Fattah 1983; Sherman et al. 1992; Tonry 2008), research has found support for the efficacy of this premise, often entailing increases in or the strategic deployment of police (Corman and Mocan 2000; Kubrin et al. 2010; Messner et al. 2007), or more severe punishment (Kessler and Levitt 1999) as means of deterring criminal

90

activity. Though, there are meaningful gaps in the literature that have left applications of deterrence concepts underdeveloped. Specifically, extant literature has devoted little attention to drug-related offending in comparison to other forms of criminality, despite the substantial portion of incarcerated persons that are drug offenders. Consequently, an often-overlooked question remains– are deterrence-based policies capable of altering an individual's rational calculus if their capacity to think clearly is distorted? More specifically, does an addict's chemical dependency compromise their ability to rationally analyze risk versus reward? These questions represent the central focus of this section.

Ultimately, among my sample, an opioid addict's worst fear is getting arrested and going to jail, though the underlying rationale is not as might be expected. The thought of being incarcerated and the subsequent existence of a criminal record might scare a non-user into obeying the law or to behave in a socially normative manner, but opioid addicts are different. They fear incarceration for another reason. Their fear, above all else, is being locked up with no access to drugs, ensuring that they will have to endure horrific withdrawals. The drive to stay well is so strong that it supplants any legal precedent, so much so that incarceration, if it were accompanied by a hypothetical and reliable supply of opioids, would be a welcomed proposition. Addicts are keenly aware of how their addiction places them at odds with the legal system, but its place in their respective mental hierarchies fluctuates and, unlike the average person, has a propensity to disappear entirely. Depending on how long they had been using, consequences that used to dissuade deviant actions, even in the smallest of ways, no longer held significance.

Deterrence Theory

Elements of deterrence theory date back as far as the 18th century to scholars such as

Cesare Beccaria (1764) and Jeremy Bentham (1789). Beccaria's work laid out a set of axioms

that sought to reform existing brutal punishment systems, arguing that they were inefficient

mechanisms of crime control. Instead, he advocated the adoption of laws that would become well

known by the citizenry and characterized by having punishment commensurate with the severity

of the offense. Bentham's work advanced this cause further, articulating his vision of punishment

as being directly linked to utilitarianism. In his view, individuals will seek to maximize personal

utility and minimize disutility as a means of contentment, creating the potential for self-

interested, anti-social behavior. From this perspective, Bentham argued the crux of social control

laid in identifying socially undesirable acts and determining a potential punishment for

performing that act that made it no longer desirable.

Deterrence theory was largely dormant until re-popularized by Becker (1968). In the

years prior, the theory had fallen out of favor, primarily due to a lack of empirical backing;

however, the economist's reintroduction of ideas closely aligning with Bentham thrust the theory

back into the scholarly discourse. Much like Bentham, Becker was focused on the role that

individual self-interest played in the decision to commit crime. Unlike other active

criminological theories of the time, Becker believed that there were no underlying criminogenic

propensities among individuals. Rather, a person will calculate the expected utility that they may

experience as the result of an action, weighing the benefit against the illegality of performing the

act.

Becker (1968) is often regarded as one of the seminal works of 20th century criminology,

having spurred extensive empirical study of his utility model, related to three common factors integral to a person's calculation: the certainty of detection, the severity of the punishment, and the celerity or swiftness of the repercussions. Early research often found negative associations between greater law enforcement activity and nearly all forms of crime, though the effects are generally regarded as modest at best (Block and Heineke 1975; Ehrlich 1972, 1973, 1975). Throughout the following years, the theory underwent expansions, focused predominantly on addressing a common criticism related to the notion of subjective perception. Contrasted against work inspired by Becker, which assumed that there were objective properties to the punishment process, studies began to account for the notion that perceptions of risk and reward varied from one individual to the next, and that the deterrent effect of potential punishments might be significantly influenced by interpersonal differences (Apel 2013; Nagin 1998; Waldo and Chiricos 1972).

Research had already examined the concept of *specific* deterrence– which holds that direct contact with the justice system dissuades a person from future offending– though, debates surrounded the greater implications of sanctions. Andenaes (1974), drawing again from Bentham (1789), sought to differentiate between specific deterrence and what he called the "general preventive effect of punishment." He argued that a key element of deterrence was that it must not only influence a given individual, but that sanctions also seek to make a crime undesirable more generally, forming of a sense of moral unity that breeds conformity. This distinction gave rise to *general* deterrence, which supposes that, assuming perfect knowledge, an individual will reason that the odds of arrest, combined with the potential consequences, will outweigh the utility of committing crimes. The popularization and differentiation between general deterrence and specific deterrence has been attributed to numerous sources (Gibbs 1975), though both variations operate under the same three core principles of certainty, severity, and celerity, at times creating overlap between them (Stafford and Warr 1993).

Later work made the effort to elaborate on these concepts further, introducing additional qualifications that more fully accounted for individual values and the role of informal sanctions (Matsueda, Kreager, and Huizinga 2006; Piliavin et al. 1986; Williams and Hawkins 1986). In one account, Sherman and colleagues (1992), drawing from a substantial body of prior research, outlined a set of consolidated hypotheses that sought to emphasized nuanced components of general deterrence. They asserted that, what Pogarsky (2002) would later label as "deterrability," depended on an individual's commitment to normative behavior. Their *conditional* hypothesis emphasized the role of shame, asserting that threats are only capable of deterring offenders who hold sufficient ties to conventional society, otherwise the stigma accompanying any sanctions will fail to matter. Second, the *replacement* hypothesis assumes that informal controls are most powerful and are responsible for preventing people from considering crime (Nagin 2013). As such, legal controls and sanctions only serve to fill the void when informal controls are absent (Matza 1964). Third, the *additive* hypothesis states that both informal and formal controls are capable of deterring potential offenders and that increases in either will increase deterrence. Ultimately, the authors' findings did not support a deterrent effect; however, they found indications of the salience of the conditional hypothesis, concluding that individuals with lower stakes in social conformity were more likely to reoffend. In this sense, individuals on the fringes of society are less likely to be influenced by the threat of sanctions, a finding that holds relevance to the study of drug-addicted persons.

Empirical assessments of deterrence have primarily focused on how police presence or the enaction of more severe sentencing influences crime rates and individuals' perception of risk.

As a whole, evidence points to a deterrent effect related to increased police presence. In a variety of localities, several studies concluded that increases in police spending and that larger police departments were associated with decreases in crime rates (Corman and Mocan 2000; Evans and Owens 2007; Levitt 1997; Marvell and Moody 1996). Others sought to take advantage of exogenous circumstances to create quasi-experimental designs, measuring the effects of increases in police presence. For example, Klick & Tabarrok (2005) examined periods of heightened terror alerts in the District of Columbia, which increased the number of officers in the field, finding a seven percent decrease in the number of daily crime reports, predominantly concentrated in property crime. As well, Levitt (1997) concluded that increases in police hiring during election years, motivated by candidates' desire to lower crime for political purposes, were successful in achieving that goal. In those years, crime rates across a number of offenses decreased anywhere from five to eight percent.

Additionally, police tactics, often focused on generating more frequent contact with the public, also appear to be capable of influencing crime rates. Although they have received considerable scrutiny for discriminatory enforcement (Alexander 2012; Murakawa and Beckett 2010), evidence has shown that proactive policing has the capability to reduce violent crime (MacDonald 2002) and overall crime rates (Kubrin et al. 2010; Sampson and Cohen 1988; Wilson and Boland 1978; Wilson and Kelling 1982). Similarly, in a review of 18 studies, Sherman (1990) found that police "crackdowns" were capable of reducing several types of crime. On an individual level, it follows that there is likely a connection between recognizing elevated police presence and changes in risk perceptions.

Several studies have shown support for specific deterrence– that an offender is more likely to perceive their probability of re-arrest to be greater when they have been punished for a past offense (Anwar and Loughran 2011; Horney and Marshall 1992; Matsueda et al. 2006; Pogarsky and Piquero 2003). Ultimately, however, crackdown measures are not a viable long-term strategy. Over time, initial deterrent effects begin to wane and continue to steadily decrease until there is only a marginal effect (Nagin 1998; Sherman 1990). It is important to note, however, that support for efficacy of increased police contact is not unanimous, with several studies finding that contact with police had no significant effect on recidivism (Nagin and Snodgrass 2013; Sherman et al. 1992).

On a larger scale, analyses of sentence enhancements have produced mixed results. A substantial proportion of this research has utilized data from California, surrounding the passage of proposition 8 in 1982 and the introduction of "three strikes" laws in 1994. With regards to the former, Kessler and Levitt (1999) concluded that legal changes produced decreases that exceeded the national average over the same period on analysis. In the case of the latter, multiple studies found at least modest support for a general deterrence effect, noting that offenders with "two strikes" recidivated at a marginally lower rate (Austin, Clark, and Hardyman 1998; Shepherd 2002). Though, Helland and Tabarrok (2007) found a more substantial effect, concluding arrest rates of two-strike offenders was reduced by roughly 20 percent. Alternatively, other studies also focused on the legal landscape of California concluded that there were no significant patterns in pre- and post-legislation crime levels (Stolzenberg and D'Alessio 1997). In fact, Webster et al. (2006) examined the work of Kessler and Levitt and found that the deterrence-related reductions in crime the authors claimed to uncover were mistaken and that decreases preceded the passage of Proposition 8.

Although there is a large amount of research examining the link between drug use and crime (Anglin and Speckart 1988; French et al. 2000; McBride and McCoy 1981), the literature documenting the relationship between drug addiction and the efficacy of deterrence is sparse. Most studies have focused on the effect of fluctuations in macro-level arrests and incarceration statistics on aggregate drug use indicators. A report issued by the PEW Charitable Trusts (2018) concluded that there was no association between state-level incarceration rates for drug crimes and self-reported drug use, drug overdose deaths, and drug arrests. As well, over a ten-year period, Friedman et al. (2011) found no significant changes in the prevalence of injection drug use associated with variations in arrest rates for the possession of heroin and cocaine. Though, importantly, the study has a number of limitations, primarily related to data availability of desirable lower-level measures, given that it analyzed the largest SMAs. A handful of studies have also drawn similar conclusions, finding that incarceration for drug offenses had no effect on recidivism rates (Mitchell et al. 2017; Perry et al. 2015).

The most developed component of the drugs and deterrence literature focuses on the deleterious consequences of proactive policing tactics. In a qualitative study of intravenous drug users in New York, Cooper et al. (2005) found that addicts were more likely to maintain injection habits and engaged in increasingly risky behavior, including the decision to reuse dirty syringes, as a result of the perceived inability to move freely because of police surveillance. Other research has consistently drawn similar conclusions, noting that increased police presence was associated with a reduced likelihood to utilize syringe exchange programs (Bluthenthal et al. 1997) and safe injection sites (Bluthenthal et al. 1999a), likely contributing to elevated risk of contracting HIV (Bluthenthal et al. 1999b), hepatitis B and C, and endocarditis (Daniels, Grytdal, and Wasley 2009; Des Jarlais et al. 2009).

Despite a lack of research focused on individual perceptions of justice contact, there is a robust literature linking opioid use with increased criminal activity. In the midst of active use, heroin addicts are between three and four times more likely to commit crimes compared to a non-drug user (Bennett, Holloway, and Farrington 2008). Similarly, others found strong, independent associations between heroin use and criminal involvement (Ball and Ross 2012; Gandossy 1980; Inciardi 1979). While there is uncertainty as to the specific reasons why these increases occur, many point to factors associated with withdrawal symptoms (Goldstein 1985) and the necessity of securing the funds to avoid them (Anglin and Speckart 1988; Cushman 1974; Gordon 1973; Lavine 1997; Senay 1999). On the surface, this interpretation makes sense, given that opioid addicts' crimes are typically non-violent offenses, such as property crime (Hunt, Lipton, and Spunt 1984) and prostitution (Kuhns, Heide, and Silverman 1992). As well, the relationship between opioid use and crime is also moderated by the extent of addicts' use. Individuals regarded as elevated users, in terms of frequency and/or volume, are more likely to commit crime at higher rates (Bennett and Holloway 2005; Hammersley et al. 1989; Kaye, Darke, and Finlay-Jones 1998), are more likely to be arrested (Farabee, Joshi, and Anglin 2001), and are more likely to be sent to prison (Turpeinen 2001).

Comprehensive research on the power of opioid-related offending has focused on changes in individual offending over time. In a review of ten studies, Hayhurst and colleagues' (2017) analysis of 27 sub-samples found that 22 yielded significant associations between crime and opioid use.[1] In each of the 22 sub-samples, participants reported committing higher levels of crime after opioid initiation compared to before their use began. Other research has also resulted in similar conclusions, finding that individual offending increases significantly after opioid initiation (Nurco et al. 1984). The inverse of this relationship has been documented as well. In a cohort study covering a three-year period, Marel et al. (2013) found that addicts' criminal involvement decreased at a significant rate following entrance into programming focused on reducing heroin use and followed a linear pattern as participants progressed through the desistance process.

Opioid Addiction and the Capacity for Rationality

There is a well-documented association between opioid use and offending. Nevertheless, the sum of extant research also reflects the lack of understanding regarding the underpinnings of this relationship. Nearly all work that exists on this subject is quantitative and many rely on macro-level aggregate predictors (Bennett et al. 2008; Boles and Miotto 2003; French et al. 2000; Hammersley et al. 1989; Inciardi 1979). This leaves a considerable gap in the literature concerning the internal processes and perception of external factors that increase an addict's likelihood of crime. The common thread uniting them remains the notion that an individual's criminal decision-making is a rational process, significantly influenced by the threat of sanction. A majority of studies have supported the efficacy of deterrence policing, though the subjective nature of risk assessment makes the prospect of applying this concept across the entire spectrum of potential offenders tenuous. Indeed, it may be the case that a would-be offender whose ability

---

[1] Of the remaining five, only one found a negative relationship (Weissman, Katsampes, and Giacinti 1974), while the others reported no statistically significant findings.

to think rationally is compromised will not perceive the risk of arrest similarly to the average

individual. Consequently, uncertainty remains as to whether deterrent effects found among larger

samples of offenders are applicable to addicts.

One proposed explanation of addicts' relationship with rationality was introduced by

Becker and Murphy's *rational addiction* model (1988). The model asserts that all addicts,

regardless of vice, are rational actors that choose to engage in activities that are deemed rational

despite accompanying consequences. While designed to apply to all addictive goods, including

caffeine and television, researchers frequently use heroin use as an example of strong negative

addictive behaviors (Kirby, Petry, and Bickel 1999; Rogeberg 2020; Verdejo-García, Alcázar-

Córcoles, and Albein-Urios 2019). At the outset, the initiation of drug use is assumed to be a

highly forward-thinking process. Before use begins, the addict-in-waiting plans the duration of

their period of heroin use in advance, assuming that they have a complete understanding of what

progressive levels of use will entail. As a negative good, heroin will simultaneously decrease a

person's baseline utility, provide gratification in the present, and increase its utility in the future,

such that it becomes increasingly important to have over time (i.e., to avoid withdrawal

symptoms). After initiating use, an individual will then weigh the pros of immediate gratification

against the cons of negative future consequences, a process that is heavily influenced by both the

chemical and psychological needs for immediate reward. In the course of this process, increased

use and potential negative side effects may outwardly appear unexpected, though, the theory

holds that this process is actually part of an addict's initial plan when use began.

Despite widespread utilization within economics, the model does not come without its

criticisms (Orphanides and Zervos 1995; Rogeberg 2020; Rogeberg and Melberg 2011). As

Laporte et al. (2017) note, there is a considerable gap between perceptions of the success of the rational addiction model and the amount of supportive empirical evidence produced. Indeed, as the authors note, many scholars acknowledge this gap and the limitations that it imposes on both theoretical development and practical policy applications (Melberg and Rogeberg 2008). For example, Orphanides and Zervos' (1998) assertion that addicts are likely to plan the duration of their use in advance, for example, to use for a year's time, is suspect. Having made this determination, an addict would then disregard the importance of time beyond that threshold, instead prioritizing only the time up until their decided end date, resulting in rash behavior. Though, the fundamental assumption in this instance places a great deal of weight on an addicts' ability to fully predict the trajectory of their use before it even begins, a premise that is at least somewhat incongruent with reality given the evidence pointing towards addicts' impulsive decision making.

While a model of this nature is well-suited for the study of innocuous vices, such as coffee (Olekalns and Bardsley 1996), movies (Sisto and Zanola 2010), or attending sporting events (Spenner, Fenn, and Crooker 2010), opioid addiction is another matter entirely. Attempts to model the individual-level thought processes and perceptions of an addict are inherently questionable, given addicts' propensity for behavioral instability. Regardless of the complexity of a proposed model, the unpredictable effects of opioid addiction are hardly reducible to a formulaic expression that is true to reality. Although the continuation of drug use or the decision to carry out drug-related crime may be deemed rational from an economic perspective, it is against the social benefit to accept its inevitability and the damages that accompany them.

The Neurological Impact of Opioids

Other disciplines have proposed alternative explanations for addicts' behavior, pointing towards the influence that chemical dependency exerts on an addict's ability to make rational decisions. The National Institute on Drug Abuse (NIDA) defines addiction as a chronic, relapsing brain disease that generates compulsive drug-seeking behavior despite negative consequences. Though contested by some (Ahmed 2010; Ahmed, Lenoir, and Guillem 2013), others have found support for the "orthodox conception of addiction," which holds that a drug addict's brain may be "hijacked" by their drug use (Heyman 2009; Pickard 2018; Satel and Lilienfeld 2013). Although the process is much more complex in a neurological sense, when a person uses heroin, receptors in the brain are flooded with dopamine, eliciting a temporary feeling of euphoria. The repetition of this process strengthens the brain's connections, reinforcing the association of drug use with euphoria (Kalivas and Alesdatter 1993). This outcome becomes especially problematic considering the enduring nature of opioid addiction. In contrast to addictions to natural sources of gratification such as food or sex, the body's desire for the effects of opioids can never be satiated, contributing to the compulsive nature of addiction (Di Chiara 2002; Wise 2002).

The desire to pursue the euphoria of opioids is an increasingly unobtainable goal. Over time, brain receptors undergo structural changes from consistent drug use (Kalivas and Alesdatter 1993). In the near term, these changes undermine the functionality of the brain's frontal subcortical circuitry, which play key roles in regulating decision-making and behavior (Fareed et al. 2017; Wang et al. 2012; Zijlstra et al. 2008). Given the novelty of the effects of the drugs, these portions of an addict's brain become hyperactive. However, over time, receptors begin to disengage, resulting in significant declines in the addict's normal mental and behavioral functionality (Goldstein and Volkow 2002, 2011).

The cognitive effects of drug-related changes in brain function are ultimately distilled to a singular outcome– a myopic focus on the procurement of drugs by whatever means necessary. Amidst the mental and physical stresses of withdrawal (Fareed et al. 2017), addicts' risk tolerance increases and is even further exacerbated as they progressively experience greater discomfort (Saddoris et al. 2015; Trifilieff et al. 2013). Consequently, throughout periods of consistent use, addicts often experience substantial decreases in their ability to accurately evaluate risk as they attempt to avoid withdrawal (Ekhtiari et al. 2017; Stewart et al. 2013, 2017). Addicts' thought processes are dominated by reflexive, impulsive decisions, most often related to a preference for immediate rewards, even at the expense of long-term consequences (Biernacki et al. 2018; MacKillop et al. 2011; Redish, Jensen, and Johnson 2008). The preoccupation with opioids also adversely affects the capacity for decision-making under ambiguous circumstances, with addicts demonstrating a reduced ability to properly process situational stimuli and make well-reasoned, proportionate decisions (Dom et al. 2006; Grant, Contoreggi, and London 2000; Loeber et al. 2009; Verdejo-Garcia et al. 2007; Vonmoos et al. 2013). Under experimental conditions, a number of studies concluded that addicts paid less attention to losses and were prone to try to "chase losses" in the face of negative feedback (Ahn et al. 2014; Fernández-Serrano, Pérez-García, and Verdejo-García 2011; Myers et al. 2016).

Further, making matters worse, addicts also tend to subvert the accumulation of negative experiences in the continuation of their pursuit of opioids, such that repeated sanctions often do not have the intended cumulative effect. These tendencies bear substantial consequences, given that addicts also typically have blunted senses of social and non-social rewards (Tobler et al.

2016), lessening their internal perceptions of the downsides associated with normatively divergent behavior such as incarceration or informal social sanctions. Unfortunately, the effects of continued exposure to chemical changes as well as other neurological damage, have the potential to last well beyond an individual's active addiction, potentially including long-term deficits in decision-making, cognitive control, and emotional blunting (Pirastu et al. 2006; Volkow, Koob, and McLellan 2016) as well as reductions in the volume of the brain's gray matter (Fareed et al. 2017; Qiu et al. 2013; Volkow, Benveniste, and McLellan 2018). These negative changes, especially among adolescents and young adults, will likely change the trajectory of a person's life, given the intensity of drug-seeking desires, which will likely interfere with normative responsibilities and increase the propensity for crime (Wang 2019).

Chapter 4. (Ir)rational Calculus: The Corruption of Risk and Reward

I was invincible. I was so concerned with getting high that at that point– the check cashing place I worked. There were like 18 fucking cameras in there. I didn't care. That's why I got felony charges working there and stealing. I knew I was going to get in trouble, but you convince yourself you won't get caught. It's one of those things you just shut off…At that moment, that's all that matters, that I was gonna be well. There was even one guy I cashed a check for. He literally took my car, went and got dope, put it in a needle for me, and passed it right over the counter there in front of the cameras. I didn't care. I did not care.

- Tiffany (WF33)

Opioid addiction wears down a person's inhibition in stages. As their use progresses, they often become increasingly indifferent to the potential legal consequences of their actions. They also become increasingly dismissive of the concrete consequences of prior contact with the justice system as well as the potential for future contact. In that sense, both general and specific deterrence largely fail to apply. While an addict is "in the stronghold," as Liz (AI.F34) called it, nothing else matters but securing the next high. Rationality ceases to exist. At best, an awareness of the law will modify an addict's approach to crime, but rarely has the ability to prevent it.

In what follows, I present three distinct stages of justice-related perceptions. First, I discuss individuals that weigh risk against reward, are aware of consequences, and modify their approach to crime in order to minimize their chances of arrest. Crime will happen in some form, but they take action to reduce risk. In this stage, the vast majority of users are still on pills, even at a high volume. The transition to the second stage often happened as an addict's means of obtaining pills was threatened. Either a script got cut off or they were unable to find or afford pills on the street. Even in the earlier stages of pill abuse, individuals experienced sickness and had an imperative to get more, but they were still capable of assessing circumstantial factors. The key differentiation being that this imperative would grow stronger over time, leading to increasingly reckless behaviors.

Second, a more advanced stage saw addicts maintain an awareness of potential justice contact but were indifferent to the consequences. Here, individuals were typically in the last moments of inconsistent pill use, resulting in frequent sickness, or had already entered into heroin abuse. As discussed in Chapter 2, there was often a point where picking up heroin "made sense" for pill addicts. Individuals in this stage viewed the prospect of arrest as an occupational hazard. Risk/reward calculations were performed, but individuals were apathetic to whatever might happen to them, effectively rendering any such calculation void. There was still a voice in their heads telling them what they were planning to do was a bad idea, but there was no scenario that would see risk outweigh reward. They had a need and pursuing it meant possible arrest. This mindset became especially common as heroin use progressed.

Lastly, the most advanced group, which was comprised solely of moderate to advanced heroin users, described a life where they failed to consider consequences in any capacity. Their daily decisions were driven solely by impulse. It was simple– need drugs, do crime. If there is an underlying maxim for opioid-related crime, it is that the greater the desperation, the greater the risk tolerance, up until the point that the concept of risk no longer applies.

Before moving to individual discussions of each of these three categories, I'm going to present Justin's story as a case examination. During the course of his opioid use, he moved through each of the three categories. Due to his extensive background in illegal activity, Justin's case provides a lengthy control period of sorts, permitting insights into the specific ways that the initiation of opioid use influenced his capacity for rationality and his perceptions of risk surrounding the decision to commit crime.

Justin

I first mentioned a bit of Justin's (WM31) story when I talked about Florida pill run operators earlier on in Chapter 1. While not directly involved, his more-than-a-decade-long career as a cocaine dealer gave him insight into colleagues' response to the burgeoning potential of organized pill collection and doctor shopping. Justin grew up as part of a family that featured several career-criminals on his stepdad's side. Predictably, he followed in their footsteps and was taught to be a "booster" (professional thief) as a young boy. His mother and his biological father, who was infrequently in the picture, both worked straight jobs and struggled to make ends meet. That outcome was not lost on Justin. The prospect of doing little work and having anything he wanted versus working hard with nothing to show for it influenced his commitment to a deviant path early,

> I was basically learning to be a booster. I would go to the stores and I didn't steal from people or anything like that, like in society. I would steal from stores. I basically had started to kind of mimic what my stepdad did. Around that time, I had started to smoke weed and I needed a way to pay for weed and I'd watched them go out stealing and I started doing what they were doing. They would compile a big ass list from people and then they would spend the day and they would go around until they rounded up everything on that list. And then that was their payday. I would go to school and do the same thing. Some people would tell me things that they wanted, or I would go to the store and I would just get a bunch of shit and I would be going to school with it.

Justin's involvement in crime as a pre-teen is contextually significant. He has actively engaged in crime for more years than he has followed the law in his life. With two decades' experience running a near-constant risk calculation, he's had ample experience to hone his craft in ways that other members of my sample did not, especially those that had no criminal involvement to speak of prior to their opioid addictions. If you've never done crime, the odds are you won't know how to do it well, especially amidst active addiction. In that sense, his eventual transition into elevated categories of arrest-related indifference is a conservative test. If anyone would have the ability to remain at the lowest, most functional level where an individual would remain cautious throughout the course of their addiction, it would have been Justin. It was engrained in him to not take unnecessary risks, yet even he was susceptible to the influence of opioids.

In the early stages of his addiction, he was capable of avoiding arrest. Before he started to use opioids, Justin was a full-time drug dealer at 17, making $6,000 in the average week. He learned the business from a family friend that had history selling cocaine. He had been active for over 30 years without getting caught. Having learned the tricks of the trade, Justin knew what red flags to look for and what he could do to cover himself as best as possible. Armed with that knowledge, he saw career potential right away, "I used to tell my cousin like, 'I'm going to sell crack for the rest of my life. Yeah, I'm going to do this rest of my life. All I got to do is answer his phone, drop this on the scales and everybody else are breaking their fucking back like mom and dad did our whole lives for nothing.' And so, I really didn't want to do anything else or be anything else after I'd started selling drugs."

In the next few years, Justin had a pair of kids, went to jail, and went to prison– both times for gun charges– and started eating percs. It started out with 5s but ramped up to 30s quickly. They were what all of his colleagues sold, so that's what he would buy, and he had the resources to buy in bulk,

> In the very beginning when I started eating 30s, everybody was going to Florida. I would buy 100, 200, 300 30s at a time…when I very first started taking 30s, I mean, I got them cheap. I could go and buy one and get it for 10, 11 bucks, or I could buy 100 of them. The first dude I was getting them from, like I said, he would charge me like 800– eight bucks a piece– but I've got people after that that would be like, "Man, if you buy 500 of them, I'll give them to you for $4 apiece, but you got to buy them from me."

With so many on hand, his habit escalated rapidly. At the peak, he found himself spending somewhere around "$1,000 to $1,300 a day on pills," and taking roughly "40 to 60 30s a day." He was able to trick himself into thinking it was harmless. He was a drug dealer– he had the money, and he had the access, and he felt great, so who's to say it was a problem?

> When my habit had progressed and progressed and progressed, I really didn't see it as progression because I never felt none of the hardships of it. Even when I spent $1,000 a day on pills, I had the money to do it and it still didn't affect my everyday life or other things that I did. I still gave my mom and them money. I still did things for other people, like nothing was going on. It was like that for years too. By the time I started thinking like, "Damn, this is a fucking problem," I had already been doing percs for eight, nine years. I'd been doing them for a while. I didn't think I was a junkie for years. I'd eat more pills in a day than most fucking people would in an entire month. And I thought that I was just okay.

He'd seen a lot of heroin addicts in his line of work, but as long as he stayed on the pills, he thought he was good. Everything was going along as it was supposed to. Even in the midst of a habit that would make a toxicologist's jaw drop, he still maintained a functional drug operation.

He wasn't dipping into his own supply and he wasn't getting arrested– he paid attention to details and was careful about who he did business with.

Where Justin differs from other opioid addicts was his immunity to the corrupting influence of pills. Many others started taking risks and stealing from big box stores when they were taking ten percent of what he did in a day. The main reason being financial capability. Not many people could afford to buy $1,000 worth of pills every day. A habit that costly necessitated some form of illegal income because it was unlikely that a person in that space would be capable of holding a straight job. Beyond that, how many people working a straight job earn that much money anyway? The proportion of those individuals that have high school educations or lower being smaller still. Justin wasn't forced to take the risks that others may have in order to secure pills. He already had an illegal income stream. However, everything changed when he transitioned to heroin.

Justin picked up heroin almost by accident. He started middlemanning for a friend that sold weight to one repeat customer in particular. Justin served as a glorified delivery man, taking a cut for himself from each drop off. Every time he went to make a delivery, the customer would chip away at him, trying to get him to try it. The customer knew that Justin was eating a large volume of percs and that they were getting harder to find. Justin was starting to be sick more often as supplies dwindled and it was beginning to interfere with his ability to conduct business, making him more amenable to a switch,

> He bought a shitload of it [heroin]. I would just go get it from one of my buddies. I would take it to him, and I'd make money off of it...Being that I got that high tolerance, he was like, "Man, if you do a couple bags of heroin, man, you'll be all right."... When I would be sick, I couldn't move. I couldn't move like I needed to. Instead of getting to somebody's house and running in, and keep things moving– I

just couldn't. Normally I'd go in, I would be giving you your dope, and I'd have two or three more orders. I'd get to the end of those orders; I'd have two or three more. I would just run and run all day. Well, when it got to that point where I can't find all the pills, I'm not moving very fast. I'm sitting in people's driveways, I'm missing money. So, the dude talked me into doing some heroin.

In Justin's words, "After I'd started doing heroin, things fucking went downhill pretty quick." Right around the same time he started heroin, his cocaine supplier was killed. He no longer had a source to get high-quality product from. It was essential to his business, otherwise his profit margins weren't where they had been previously, and he wouldn't be able to make it stretch as far when he went to prepare it for sale. In the past, a situation like this was fixable. It had happened before, several years ago, but being on heroin changed how the situation played out, "Once I started doing heroin…My thought process wasn't the same. And if I would've never started doing heroin, I could've thought myself out of that situation. There had been, over the years of being on pain pills, I had a lot of situations that happened like that and I'd just dealt with them. When shit like that would happen, you just got to deal with it." His business suffered and over the course of the next year he would lose his clientele due to his rising personal addiction.

There was something different about heroin. It was messing with his mind. He knew it. He noticed it constantly. Suddenly, there was a sense of desperation that he'd never felt before. Justin made a lot of money selling drugs, but a crucial part of his operation was making sure he had enough money to re-up, using a large portion of his profits to buy more at wholesale prices to then break down, repackage, and sell,

> Heroin gives you an opioid high, but there's something fucking different about it,
> I don't know what it is. All those years that I'd done pills, I did have some control
> over it. Even when I'd done a lot...just for instance of how the transition happen,
> you think about what I'm doing. I'm selling drugs. I have thousands of dollars in

my pocket, but it was re-up money. So, I'd be fucking sick. When that transition
actually happened and I started doing heroin, that shit didn't fucking matter
anymore. I didn't care. There was just something psychologically different about
the drug.

A wholesaler prioritizes selling a substantial volume of a product at a lower price, the upside

being avoiding hundreds of micro-transactions. If Justin didn't have a large sum of money, they

wouldn't give him a price that ensured adequate profit margins. Heroin was throwing everything

off track.

When he could no longer re-up and he'd spent all of his money on heroin, Justin became

increasingly desperate. Previously, in all of the years he was using pills and remained in stage

one, he was making the same risk/reward calculations he'd been making his entire life– he just

had an addiction while he was doing it. He was aware of risks and took steps to minimize them

as much as possible. In the early stages of heroin use, he started stealing more often, but still had

a sense of what carried more risk and how to avoid it. Specifically, he maintained a sense of the

crimes that he would and would not do,

> I would always do risk, "What am I going get [as punishment] for what I'm
> doing? Is it worth what I'm doing, or can I do something easier?" I did always
> think about stuff like that…I wouldn't do an armed robbery. I wouldn't do a home
> invasion or something like that because there's just so much more risk and stuff as
> to, not only if you get caught, are you're going to go to jail, but on the other side
> of it. Even if you never got caught by the police, if I was to rob you, come into
> your house, anything like that– I could have to kill you or get killed
> myself…versus you're a roofer, I'm breaking into your van sitting on the street,
> and take everything out of it and make pretty good chunk of money.

He was going to go do crime, that was a guarantee. He was sick. Still, his brain worked. As his

use worsened, that stopped being the case,

The fact I didn't have the money to pay for the drugs that I did and after all that time of having the money to buy whatever I want and things like that, your tolerance is outrageous. So, I would do crazy shit. I'd be going out stealing and be getting caught. I'd be getting caught at the stores boosting, fucking going out stealing people's shit, getting pulled over, going to jail. Once I started having to do shit like that, I'd go to jail all the damn time…For instance, I got caught stealing out here at Lowe's. Going to hardware stores and stealing was the easiest thing in the world– when you go and do that, you got the machine that buys the gift card back for 65%. Back in the day, you used to have to go, steal shit, return it, get the gift card because you don't got a receipt. And then take the gift card and find somebody to buy it…I mean, if I get caught, I get caught.

Justin had entered stage two. He was aware that what he was doing carried risk. He was calculating risk/reward, but counter to what theory would predict (Becker 1968), it wasn't impacting his actions in any way. Knowing there was a high probability of getting caught no longer mattered and getting arrested and spending time in jail had no effect on him. It was essentially getting put in timeout for a few days or weeks at a time. In the time immediately preceding a crime, Justin was arriving at different conclusions when he contemplated taking illegal action,

I wasn't necessarily like constantly worried, but yeah, you'd get nervous about things and I'd wonder "Am I going to fucking caught doing this?" Once you start getting into so much of drug use, you know that your thought process doesn't work right. So, you might still do a risk assessment of what you're doing, and you might think it's the same as when you wasn't getting high, but it's not. Risk assessment before you're using would be a breakdown, every single part in this. After years of using drugs, I would know that that's happening to me. I would be thinking, just thinking about things, not be able to work out a plan. It's like you're just stuck. Something that would be simple that you know that you used to be able to do. It was just gone. After using, you think it's the same type of thing, but the risk assessment is "Are there any fucking cops in here? No? Let's go. It's in there and we need it."…Before drug use, I would commit a lot more crimes that made a lot more money, that I got caught for way less…Boosting is the simplest thing in the world. When I was younger, I did that shit all the time. I did get caught here and there, but not like after I got older and was on drugs. It was like I'd go into stores and had a sign that said "thief" on me. I swear to God, man.

Justin was deep into stage two. He wasn't capable of properly formulating an accurate assessment of risk versus reward. He still cared about risk to a certain extent, but it paled in comparison to what he had done for years. It was limited to his immediate surroundings, and even then, was only a momentary thought. It was never the case that he would see a police officer and decide to pack it up and go home.

Eventually, Justin got worse and progressed to stage three. As expected, the higher his use got, the greater his focus on avoiding withdrawals became (Ekhtiari et al. 2017). He stopped bothering to even think about risk. His illegal activity was reduced to pure impulse, borne out of perceived life and death necessity, "If I was going out stealing, it wouldn't matter what I was stealing. I wouldn't think about, 'Well, if I get caught, man, this is what's going to happen.' You don't think about none of that stuff ever. You just go and you just do what you got to do." Ultimately, there was documentation to back up his views. Before it was all said and done, Justin was arrested more than 40 times for drug-related crimes during the course of his heroin addiction. Clearly, the arrests didn't have any effect on his desire to commit crime; he became more brazen over time and the prospect of enhanced punishment was a hollow threat. The needle became the only thing that mattered to him anymore.

Given the sheer volume of his arrest record, I asked him if the kind of charges he received mattered, or if the threat of doing a longer sentence would have dissuaded him in any way, he replied, "If they change the laws around on it, I really don't think that it's going to make much of a difference. If you make a felony a misdemeanor or make a misdemeanor a felony, none of that's going to matter because the way the addict is going to think about it, you don't care."

Stage One: Fear of Arrest and the Alteration of Actions

> *It was the cat and mouse game, catch me if you can. I'm not going to get caught doing it this way to support my habit…If I'm going to commit a crime, is it worth doing the time for that crime? Definitely, yeah. If you think about that, the felonies, like– I'm not going to go kill somebody for some dope. I'm not going to go put anybody in harm's way for some dope. But I'll do something stupid for dope. There's definitely a line, I just don't know what it is, but the little petty crimes didn't really scare me.*
>
> *- Henry (WM30)*

Like Justin, Henry knew he was going to commit a crime. He was sick, broke, and needed money. Rather than experience withdrawals, he had to go make something happen. In his case, his go-to was petty theft. His thought process was hijacked by opioids to an extent, but he maintained a semblance of agency (Pickard 2018). He knew better than to walk into the nearest store, load up, and run. Instead, he picked his targets to minimize the chances that he would be detained. In that sense, members of this first category were conducting some form of a risk/reward calculation and then *altering* their behaviors. He was well aware of the risks that his plan still entailed, lamenting that there was only so much he could do to insulate himself beyond targeting specific stores. When I asked him if there was anything he did to reduce the chances of getting caught while in the act, he responded, "Not really, I would just...if I was boosting or stealing, I would just be as smart as possible about it. You know? It just made me more cautious, because I didn't want to go to jail and be dope sick."

Henry is a quintessential case of an early-stage opioid-addicted offender. Avoiding sickness, and, in particular, avoiding being sick in jail, was his number one priority. He had a singular focus, but he knew that being reckless had consequences– just not the ones that lawmakers intended. To be clear, he did not fear having a record and he only feared being incarcerated in that it would prevent him from getting high, a commonality he shared with nearly every person in my sample.

An opioid-addicted brain does not function properly. An addict's ability to consider consequences and act accordingly based on norms surrounding deviant behavior are out the window. They know what they are doing is wrong, but they are indifferent. They care only as much to attempt to avoid arrest.

When she was deep into her pill addiction, Tamika (BF29) also consistently relied on stealing as her main source of income to pay for perc 30s. After getting away with it several times, she believed she had developed a system that she thought aided her ability to evade detection, "It became a job [theft]…I didn't care. I felt like I was a professional. I was going every day; it was a nine-to-five. I would literally get up, get dressed, go. I even had costumes. It was crazy." Tamika was also selective in her approach once she was inside a store and took care to keep track of the goods she stole,"…everything I always did, I made sure I never got a felony– $1,000 is considered a felony. I never got to a felony because, I don't know, people look at felons a whole lot different…some people might look over misdemeanors. If you have felonies, you really can't do anything. I always made sure it was no felony. I cared about a little bit of something but didn't care about much." By dressing in a certain way, combined with staying below a certain dollar threshold, Tamika was still assessing risk/reward. Although she notes not caring about the notion of getting caught in a general sense, her modified actions indicate some change in behavior based on perceptions of risk.

Jennifer (WM31), like Tamika, relied heavily on retail theft as the main source of illegal income to feed her addiction. Her actions were also heavily influenced by the perceived necessity of avoiding being sick, especially in jail. To improve her odds of escape, she would develop a strategy that she believed would increase the likelihood of successfully evading detection,

> I was pretty confident, but I used to think that I was smart about it. I did a good cat and mouse kind of game when I was in the stores and stuff and I feel like that gave me a little advantage because I would know how to lure them away from the doors so I could get out. It was just something– I had to be smart or else I wasn't getting high that day…If you get caught, you're going to jail sick and that's the worst feeling you can ever go through. You never want to be in jail sick. You never want to be in jail, but definitely not sick.

Avoiding arrest wasn't about a moral opposition to receiving sanctions; rather, incarceration guaranteed that she was going to go be forced to white-knuckle her inevitable withdrawals. Even as a free woman, Jennifer faced a similar fate if she did not steal on a given day. She was going to be sick. Worse, as her sickness progressed, she would become a less capable thief, making it even harder to get away with crime.

Nick (WM43) was also aware of the risk that stealing carried. When he first began to commit crime to fuel his addiction, he targeted homes. After several successful burglaries, he recognized that he was exposing himself to unnecessary danger. There were alternatives that could potentially be as lucrative, but would carry lesser risk of being caught in the act,

I used to break into homes where people lived in, but then I stopped breaking in
and I started breaking into houses where they were rehabbing the houses and they
leave tools and materials. They would only be a F4, F5. So, if I did get caught, I
wouldn't go to prison for as long. I justify it like that. As long as they don't catch
your ass for a three, two, or one, I'm okay. I felt like I wasn't really harming
anyone even though it was because it was stuff that I was taking, but I didn't feel
like I was like traumatizing nobody.

By stealing from construction areas, usually at night, the probability of encountering another person was drastically reduced. There was never a time that Nick considered not stealing; he maintained the same risk tolerance, but he was analyzing his situation enough to recognize a better opportunity. The driving force behind Nick's change in strategy was risk avoidance, but it was also about self-perception. Like many others in the earlier stages of addiction-related crime, Nick did not have a history of criminal activity prior to his addiction. The things that he found himself doing, like burglarizing homes, was counter to how he used to think of himself. Revising his actions to focus on "victimless" crimes helped resolve the conflict he felt between his past sense of self and his present actions.

Ryan (WM49) also contended with changing self-perceptions as his addiction-related crime increased. He began using the pills as a result of a work-related construction accident and after years on them– he was taking double-digit perc 30s per day– his prescription was halted. His legitimate income could no longer cover the cost, so he turned to property crime as well,

I knew what the risk was. I knew that there was a possibility of getting caught.
But in my mind, I figured that I had a good plan, I'm smart enough. I can get away
with it. "I'm smart enough to do this." It's not this rash, like, "I'm going to go stick
up a liquor store," or something like that. I had a value system as I was raised.
You don't steal, you don't deceive people. Be honest with them and treat others
how you want to be treated yourself. That's how I was raised, but I was in full-

blown addiction, not really caring about others. Everything was about me, and what I wanted. How I was going to get it, and not concerned with other's feelings, or how it affected them really.

Ryan knew he was an addict, but he wasn't so far-gone that he couldn't juxtapose two options and pick the one with less risk, contrasting his own plans against those of an impulsive stick-up artist demonstrates that capability. In his mind, planning out his crimes in advance gave him the ability to leverage his intelligence to avoid the greatest degree of risk possible. As well, like Nick, it's clear that Ryan was dealing with internal moral conflict. In a manner very similar to individuals that made deals with themselves about "moving the lines" regarding heroin use, Ryan's comparison of his actions with a crime he thought was more severe than what he'd go on to commit helped him preserve his sense of being a "good" person caught up in a bad situation, rather than facing his new reality.

Stage Two: The Acknowledgment and Rejection of Risk

> *Yeah, I was afraid. But that didn't stop me from doing it. My fear of being sick overrode my fear of going to jail. Even though when I went to jail, I would be sick. My fear of being sick in that moment took precedent over anything and everything else, no matter who I was around, where I was at. It didn't matter. I think about the shit that I'm doing, I think about the repercussions and the shit that I can have from it, and consequences. But it doesn't deter me from still doing them.*

> *- Kelly (WF27)*

Sickness. The desperation that it induced in an addict is unlike any pressure they'd experienced before in their lives. The transition to the second stage of risk/reward calculation most often aligned with an addict's first true dry spell, whether it was due to incarceration, poverty, or scarcity, they couldn't get what they needed for an extended period of time. Sickness was something addicts in stage one had been exposed to, but most hadn't yet felt its full force. Perhaps they had fewer pills than they'd needed in those times– but they had *something* in the span of a few days. They would be sick, sure, but not feeling like they were edge-of-dying sick. When they finally did reach that point, their recognition of risk held no sway on what they would do next. Such was the case with Joel (WM35),

> I was always worried about getting caught, especially after getting arrested a couple of times. But when you're withdrawing, you're not really thinking about if I get caught, you're thinking I've got to get away with this. The withdrawals, it's the worst feeling in the world. Worse than any flu I've ever had. It scares a lot of people, and you've got to go out there and do what you've got to do before they start, because when they start– I couldn't do nothing. I was begging, borrowing, stealing off of whoever…it's not really thinking "I could go to jail for this," it's "I could get $100 for this." Pretty much the only thing you're thinking about if you get caught is how sick you're going to be in jail.

Without the funds to support a well-developed heroin habit, he became desperate, increasing his risk tolerance while simultaneously decreasing his fear of arrest (Anglin and Speckart 1988; Cushman 1974; Lavine 1997). It was the feeling of being backed into a corner. He and his wife both got on it and slowly lost everything. At that stage, crime became a necessity, because avoiding sickness felt like it was a life and death ordeal.

Dale's (WM28) family lived deep in the country, but they decided to move to the worst neighborhood in the city when he was 19. Up until then, he'd never even seen any kind of drugs. He started smoking weed off and on with friends he'd made. It was constantly around. Dale got sucked into opioids from one of those friend's sure-fire remedy for the abscess in his mouth that was so painful it made it impossible to sleep. Once pills no longer got him high, he developed a consistent heroin habit and got involved selling drugs to cover the expense. He was middlemanning for dealers and was making decent money, but his habit was becoming increasingly costly. When it became hard to conceal his use, he was cut out of the operation, "I would fuck up the money or now nobody wants to work with me because they know I'm doing heroin, so they're not trying to sell me heroin no more. It started slowing on down and then I don't have no heroin. Now what I am I going to do? I'm doing criminal shit like breaking into cars, breaking into houses, and robbing people." Without the money from selling, Dale got desperate. When he was middlemanning, but before he graduated to heroin, he was careful. He trusted the guys that he worked for and only made deals with people that could be vouched for. There's always a risk of getting caught for drug possession or distribution, but he made sure he took steps to minimize it. He no longer had that luxury. His body demanded dope, causing him to act more rashly, often for smaller rewards (Tobler et al. 2016). He was aware of what he was doing, but he felt as if he had little choice, "I was taking a lot more risks with the crimes that I was committing. Not thinking them out. Doing them with people that I wasn't close with, that I didn't really know, didn't really know the situation I was getting myself into, but like I said, I figured it was worth the risk because I needed to maintain my addiction." He continued, "I didn't give a fuck. A part of me would get scared to get picked up because I don't want to go to jail dope sick. I would go by any means to get dope. I didn't give a fuck about getting caught. I just didn't want to go dope sick."

Many found themselves in similar positions. While their respective progressions into stage two did not perfectly overlap with their first severe withdrawal episode, most had graduated to heroin. As those addictions progressed, it was inevitable at one time or another that they would go without and experience withdrawals. Whenever that took place, it left an indelible mark. What they felt in that moment was seared into their minds, underscoring just how important it was that they never have to go through what they just had ever again. Consequently, going forward, it drove them to do whatever it took to get dope.

Nicole (WF26), for example, was well aware that stealing from stores would be dangerous, but it didn't matter, "I felt like it would be risky, but I would still do it. It wasn't this complicated thing. It was just, 'I need to get well. I can't right now, I got to go do what I got to do.'" Similarly, Jessica (WF35) described feeling a sense of helpless obligation, "For me, getting arrested was always an underlying fear. But it was like, I couldn't be sick. I would do whatever I had to do. So as much as I thought about getting caught, I just hoped that I didn't get caught, because there were times where I did...I did a lot of illegal things." Criminal record accumulation notwithstanding, nothing was more important than avoiding being sick. Rachel (WF28) was also scared, but, ultimately, it did not matter because the need to get high, once again, effectively nullified the process of weighing risk versus reward, "You are scared. I'm scared of it [arrest]. But the power of that heroin just negated all that. I didn't care. I was just like...I was willing to take the risk of getting in trouble just to get a little high." Eventually, even for people with spotless legal backgrounds like Stephanie (WF31), heroin became their top priority and getting arrested didn't matter, "I didn't care. I didn't wanna be sick. I've always worried about getting in trouble my whole life. I don't know why, but I didn't care. I felt like the way I was doing it wasn't as risky, and it's definitely risky now I say it out loud."

The increased sense of urgency that opioid users felt during the second stage of addiction had a cumulative effect. The commission of criminal acts that carried greater risk took a mental toll. It's not as if they were completely devoid of thought or were immune to what was transpiring– that came later, in stage three. Everyone in stage two knew what they were doing but they were so worn down by the daily, and even hourly grind of chasing dope that all they could muster was apathy.

> I knew every single thing I did as an addict had consequences; I just didn't care. I didn't care because I really, literally, my entire day consisted of me waking up, rolling off the couch, getting high, and then figuring out how I'm going to get high two hours later and so on and so forth…I would worry about being arrested and I'd be worried to death and I'd be shaking when I got back in the car after I jumped out of a window or whatever, I'd be shaking because I know I'd been this close to being caught but I didn't get caught.

Jennifer (WF31) arrived at a place where the risk of getting caught was part of a miserable routine that demanded her attention and faithful adherence. Her pattern of cyclical behavior had become a survival mechanism, used to cope with both the physical and mental strain caused by her worsening conditions.

For everyone at this stage, staying well engendered a sense of need that overrode any risk they knew they were inviting upon themselves. They all mentioned fear or risk, but also unanimously ignored it because it was an obstacle to getting high and staying well. Risk and reward were still fighting one another in their minds, but risk had both arms tied behind it's back– there was no circumstance where it was going to come out on top. While many do not explicitly mention having a warped calculation process, their views on the necessity of their actions demonstrate its presence and its salience.

Others articulated process of their changing risk/reward calculus in more detail. For Jacob (WM39), altering it was a key part of making peace with what he was doing. Taking large risks was such a common occurrence that it started to lose meaning; he became numb to its significance. It remained a constant presence in his mind, but his heroin habit did not permit him to redirect to a path that carried less risk,

> I know that it destroys or upsets the risk/reward system in your head, so you're going to take bigger risks for less reward. I know that. I know that my perception was changed…I'm going in bad neighborhoods…I knew that it was risky. I knew that people carry guns. I've had to carry guns. I know that things happen. I know that people get robbed, but it never happened to me…being a part of the subculture is like cops and robbers. It's part of life. Again, it's just…they got a job to do and so do we.

When Jacob was on pills, he was careful. He always tried to buy them through people that he knew and trusted. Once he transitioned to heroin, everything changed. Suddenly he was taking more risks. He was middlemanning more often, more recklessly. Part of that meant a greater descent into criminal life, but it was a necessity to stay well, so he developed the ability to turn off his reservations.

Stage Three: Impulse

> *When you get high, you don't think about getting caught. You don't think, "Oh, I'm selling dope. Oh, I might get 20 fucking years." You just do it, you know? You don't think. Addicts don't think, we just do. We act on impulse. We don't think at all.*
>
> *- Robin (W.TW27)*

Individuals were capable of worse, and stage three was the worst that it got. For some, not only was rationality out the window– thinking itself became an inconvenience. Doing whatever had to be done to get high became daily life. Heroin addiction was behind the wheel and advanced-stage addicts were merely passengers. For Todd (WM36), consequences were afterthoughts,

> It was always act first and deal with the bullshit later. When you're getting high on this shit [heroin] all you're doing is looking at the here and now. You aren't looking down the road at all 'cause you're in survival mode. It's just going one high, to the next, to the next, and the next, to the next. Literally, your body needs that to be well. That's pretty much the only thing on your mind. All the other crimes and the shit that comes with it? It's all to keep yourself from feeling like death.

Every action that Todd took, illegal or otherwise, was only concerned with the present. He no longer had the capacity to assess a situation and determine the risk that it posed to him, let alone alter his behavior to minimize his chances of arrest. His heroin use ensured that his withdrawal symptoms would feel like a near-death experience– he'd been there before– but his rising tolerance also meant that he required increasingly large amounts of the drug to fend off sickness. Over time, his finances depleted, making him become bolder as the price tag for his daily dope bill continued to rise.

The "whatever it takes" attitude ensures tunnel vision. Like Todd, Kevin (WM23) arrived at the same destination. He gradually dealt with the movement of his personal "lines" regarding the acceptability of heroin use. By the time he crossed the last line and started shooting heroin, his sense of right and wrong or risky and safe dissipated. His thinking became compartmentalized. If he was sick, or knew he was going to be sick, he was focused solely on the present, "All I was looking at was what was right in front of me at that point in time…It just kind of got real narrowed down to where I wasn't thinking about what the long-term effects of this were going to be on me. It was a minute-by-minute, hour-by-hour type of way of living where I was not focused on anything except for what can I do in order to sustain my habit."

During stage three, addicts became so myopic that even the *certainty* of arrest wasn't a deterrent. Raquel (BF42) was one of the individuals that described falling into this mindset, "I want it. I'm going to do it [crime] and that's what I'm gonna do. I really didn't give a fuck. You could see that a person would set me up. I would still do it knowing that within a couple hours I'm going to get caught. Not even days away, but it was that important for me to get what I wanted at that moment." Over time, Raquel had moved through the gears. Her use started with pills, got heavier, transitioned to heroin, and then that got heavier too. For the longest time, the stigma of heroin led her to conceal her use from friends and family at all costs. By the time she reached stage three, she was so far gone that everyone knew she was using, and she didn't even care anymore. The drug had its hooks so deep that the damage that she did, and all of the arrests she'd accumulate, didn't make her flinch.

After several years on dope, Mason (WM32) was in a similar position by the time he'd lost everything. He and his girl each developed a $300 per day pill habit before they made the switch to heroin. They were broke and $20 per day just made sense. Their resources were depleted from trying to stay well on pills, but heroin offered a means of actually getting high again for the first time in years. They both started out snorting it and when that wasn't working, they smoked it. When child services took their kids, Mason left her after she began prostituting. Alone, he started shooting dope. It didn't take long to get to the darkest of places, wishing he wouldn't wake up each time he pushed down the plunger. He had been an active dealer nearly up until he started shooting it. He was letting others trap out of his house, a move that prompted the drug raid that took his kids. He pushed into stage three soon thereafter and daily life became a

Bill Murray-esque Groundhog's Day cycle of wake up, do something unbelievably stupid for dope money, and do it all over. Like Raquel, getting caught wasn't on his mind. There was no more risk versus reward. His eye was always on the prize,

> I used to not think about the consequences. I just worried about what I could get right now. Down the road, I'll worry about that when I get there. I'm trying to get through right now…I never cared. I never really gave a shit. When I was in active addiction, that drug was number one. I don't care if I'm on camera, whatever. Because being scared...If I'm scared, I'm not going to get high. You know what I mean? I was really careless and stupid. It started off me being careful, but once I got to the point where I started shooting it and I got used to committing crimes and shit, then it was like fuck everything…there was no limit to what I'd do out there.

Mason stayed in the earlier stages of risk perception for over eight years. Pills were plentiful and cheap for the majority of that time, which kept him from being too careless. After he transitioned to heroin the withdrawals pushed him to the doorstep of stage three as his tolerance rose, only to take the last step once his kids were gone. He'd been arrested many times before, so being on camera guaranteed a warrant even if he escaped the scene. He didn't care.

Patrick's (WM44) version of stage three was similar to Mason's. Impulse and apathy dictated everything he did. By the time he'd gotten deep into heroin use, his ability to assess risk was long gone. It just didn't register anymore,

> I don't know how I didn't get caught. I would be like– I didn't care. When you don't care, you don't get caught. I didn't care if there's cameras. I would steal anything. I'm an opportunist when I'm out there. If it's available, I'm gonna take it. I've always went to rich neighborhoods. If a garage is open or something like that, grab something. That's what I did. But right now...I can't even think of fucking

stealing a Monster drink from a gas station. Can't do it. Today, when I'm clean, I
don't steal. I work.

It became simple– see object, steal object. He wouldn't bother to see if someone was in the
garage; if it were open, he was going in and he was leaving with something he could sell. Heroin
had elevated his desire for immediate rewards so greatly that he disregarded situational stimuli,
as expected in advanced addicts (Dom et al. 2006; Grant et al. 2000; Loeber et al. 2009; Verdejo-
Garcia et al. 2007; Vonmoos et al. 2013). There was no thought of taking precautions. Even a
security camera wasn't going to get in the way of him making sure he stayed well. Contrasted
against who he is today, getting back to the person he was before opioids, it becomes clearer how
powerful heavy heroin addiction can be. It took Patrick so far out of his character that he
couldn't fathom doing a fraction of what he was willing to do to avoid being sick.

Christine (WF26) had used drugs before she started using opioids, but none of those took
hold of her life or changed her like heroin did. She grew up in a rural area where there wasn't
much else to do but drink or get high. She started smoking weed at 13 and tried meth, coke, and
crack before she was 17. She was sexually assaulted as a teenager, combined with several
relocations, an alcoholic mother, and constant trips in and out of foster care, she endured a lot of
trauma as a teenager and drugs helped. She had kids of her own by 20 and making sure she was a
present mother was important to her. She'd never had that. Percs weren't big where she was
living, but the first time she received a script at 17 from her C-section, she fell in love, "I tell you
what, when I first did a perc, I loved it. I loved it. It just, I was going through a lot with having
my son and his dad. He was just cheating on me and doing some things, so when I took that
Percocet, it really numbed me. It made me feel good." She stayed on the pills for several years
and was able to get scripts for made up ailments, so she always had a supply. She lost her job and

her scripts, so she started selling. She used percs when she could, but rarely had as much as she would have liked. Then, a close friend offered Christine heroin when she complained of a toothache, "Long story short, I went over to his house one night for a toothache, and he gave me some heroin. After that, it just got more and more and more and more. As soon as I shot it, it just...It was never-ending." Soon after, she moved into stage three. She got reckless with selling and everyone knew who she was. It was an open secret and those attract attention from law enforcement. It wasn't just the selling anymore either. Christine expanded into any crime that she could. There was no more planning things out– if an opportunity presented itself, she acted on it,

> It seemed like when I did the heroin, that's when everything got worse…I started ripping off people, breaking in houses. Just all kinds...It really took me down…It escalated…When you do heroin, and you get on that needle, it's just like fuck everything and everybody. I robbed and stole and did anything and everything. It took me out of my character. I don't feel like crack took me out of my character as much as heroin did.

Christine had been on crack consistently for at least four years before she was an opioid addict, so she had ample experience to appreciate the differences between them. On crack, she was still able to be a mom, hold a job, and was able to conceal her use. On heroin, that all changed. Just as Patrick had, she became an opportunist. If she had a chance to make dope money, she was going to do it, regardless of what it entailed.

Prior to getting into opioids, Melissa (WF34) had no criminal record. When she was a teenager, she had a bout with ecstasy addiction, but that lasted less than a few months. From that point on, she lived a fairly normal life. She had a husband, a few kids, a job, and a home, but things turned sour when she got hooked on percs. Her husband had a pill habit that went back several years that he'd kept secret. He was abusive, controlling, and weaponized addiction to bring her closer to him. In his mind, her growing addiction that he cultivated made it more difficult for her to leave. When Melissa was in stage one, she limited her crimes to the least severe charges possible and always acted with an abundance of caution. When the couple lost custody of their kids, she pushed into stage two. Her husband was always a negative influence when it came to the extent of her criminal activity, but as her life worsened, she found herself caring less about his manipulation and the risk she was exposed to. Out of necessity, they transitioned to fentanyl. Predictably, it didn't take long to progress into the final stage.

Looking back on her addiction, Melissa was mortified at the lengths she would go to ensure she stayed well. The level of indifference and desperation that she developed went far beyond earlier stages of addiction. In hindsight, she hardly believed how differently she assessed risk,

> In the beginning when I was on pills, yes, I was afraid to get caught. Once I started fentanyl, I didn't give a shit. To me it was, I thought I was superwoman. I didn't think… Before, I would always try to find a way to not get myself caught, pre-plan ahead. When you're sick on fentanyl you aren't pre-planning shit. It just happened. Early on, I never wanted to be a felon. I went 33 years of my life without even having– all I had was a speeding ticket. I didn't want to be a felon and that's what my charge was…On Percocet, if they would've said "You're going to have a felony or you've got to stop taking Percocet," I would've stopped taking the Percocet because I didn't want to get the felony. Again, that fentanyl is something crazy. And you just don't give a shit what you are doing or who you're doing it to. When I was on fentanyl, you could have told me, "Hey, get off the fentanyl or you're going to have a felony." I would have been like, "All right. Of what degree?"…I don't think I would have cared how long I got locked up. Honestly, I really don't. Now when I was on the pills, yes. On the fentanyl, no. It's a whole different ball game. I promise you.

When an addict is as far gone as Melissa was, there's little that can be done legally to dissuade them from doing whatever they need to do to get high. As she indicated, her escalation to fentanyl was the point of no return. Had she been threatened with consequences when she was on pills, it may have mattered to her. She was likely still "deterrable" at that stage (Pogarsky 2002). Before, her traditional family life was something she was proud of. It was only after the hard opioids entered the picture that it started to no longer matter. We'll never know for sure, but taken at face value, there may have been a window where she could have been redirected to a better course.

Randy (WM35) provided yet another example of an individual in stage three that demonstrated a stark contrast between who he was while in active heroin addiction, compared to who he was, and is now, when he's not using,

> Consequences never ran through my head. It was always one track, one mission. Don't care what happens. I'm doing it. I'll give you an example: I drove 20 minutes at 3:00 in the morning with no headlights to get dope. Who cares if I get pulled over? Who cares if I kill somebody? Driving around all the fucking time 3:00 in the morning in the city, to the worst neighborhood in the city, all the way back around and was determined. That's how strong my disease is. I mean, that's insane. I want to get high. And I wasn't even sick at that point. I just wanted to keep going. So, that's the kind of insanity it does to you. I won't even drive down the street to get cigarettes if my freaking tag light's out now. You know what I mean? I had a car sitting in my driveway for three months and wouldn't drive it because I just didn't have my license back. It's just a complete black and white difference.

Now, think what he would have been willing to do if he had been sick– there's truly no limit when someone like Randy reaches the apex of shooting dope.

Chapter 5. Examining the Efficacy of Justice Contact: The Consistent Cycle of Arrest, Release, and Relapse

I had like 30 drug arrests. I didn't give a fuck. Getting dope sick, get clean, get back out, and go do it again. I had that same mentality every time. It didn't matter what the consequence was. It didn't matter how much time I had to go do. It was the same song and dance when I got back out. Or when I went to jail. I didn't care. I didn't care how long I had to go to jail for, whether it was 30 days, or any day, six months. When I got out, I want to do the same damn thing.

- Keith (WM45)

There is little ambiguity– the deeper an addict gets into opioid use, the less likely they are to be dissuaded by the threat of legal consequences. This reality casts doubt on the efficacy of general deterrence in this case (Andenaes 1968; Meier and Johnson 1977). However, even in the absence of the fear of arrest, there may be hope that the effect of justice interaction may serve as a catalyst for change. Unfortunately, in practice, this was not the case. With relation to opioid addicts, the problem with punishment is that it's an ineffective solution for the problem it seeks to address. Spending time behind bars, at its core, cannot force an addict to decide they are done using. The deeper a person went into opioid addiction, the more likely they were to have stopped caring about the prospect of another arrest, even once they had ventured into double-digit trips inside.

Often, addicts had a propensity to use within the first day of release from any given period of incarceration, demonstrating that time served often did not have the intended reformative impact. Nothing was going to stand in addicts' way of getting what they wanted, even the prospect of returning to a jail cell. While incarceration was frequently successful at forcing addicts through the cycle of withdrawal, as their release date drew near, it became clear that enduring that process did little beyond causing discomfort. This finding is counter to the hopes and expectations of a justice system that frequently relies upon incapacitation as a mechanism to reduce future offending (Alexander 2012; Garland 2001; Gottschalk 2006, 2006), necessitating further investigation into the implications these findings have for the policing of addicts. Here, I'll detail addicts' experiences with arrest and incarceration and how they influenced their respective desires to continue using opioids.

Same Song and Dance: Right Back to Using

In exceptionally rare cases, incarceration was the wake-up call that it was intended to be. Even then, incarceration was only one piece in a much larger puzzle. The vast majority of the time, however, incarceration was nothing more than a glorified time out. In effect, the state had pushed the pause button on an addict's mission to use. The intended significance of the experience failed to register with them in any lasting way. To a sober, law-abiding individual, spending time in jail is likely going to cause a beneficial correct to deviant behavior; however, they have the benefit of not being an opioid addict.

For advanced users, the progression of a one-track, reward-driven way of thinking gives them the capability to overlook present conditions. Incarceration is merely an impediment to getting well. Even after enduring the entirety of withdrawals while locked up, addicts don't forget. Their one true love is waiting for them on the outside and they're going back to it as soon as humanly possible, regardless of what stands in their way. Such was the case with Nick (WM43), whose time inside was spent obsessing over the getting well and how badly he wanted it again, "Just the regular withdrawal symptoms. I get sick, no energy, sweating, diarrhea, curled up on the floor, can't eat…It probably lasted like 14 days and then I did it all over again…I was just ready to get out and do it again. Besides, I have to think about it because while I was in there, it's all I could think about it and I was like, 'I'll get some [heroin] when I get home.' I started getting high again instantly." Whether he was using, clean, incarcerated, or free, Nick was too preoccupied with copping again that present circumstances were irrelevant. The only effect that incarceration had was as a temporary delay to the next time a needle went in his arm. He didn't stop after the other times he was forced to get clean, either. Instead, with each lock-up, he sharpened his focus on what he desired most.

Given the strength of addicts' indifference to consequences, it's not surprising there were a lot of people like Nick. Jennifer (WF31) also recalled the misery of withdrawing in jail, but similarly noted that it did little but cause momentary discomfort. She knew she was going to use as soon as she got out,

> I laid there, I detoxed, I hated it. I hated every second of it. I didn't eat, I didn't drink, I just laid there and pretty much died the whole time I was there until I started feeling better and then I'd get out and then I do the same fucking thing. Go out and get high. I'd have my mom drive me and be like, "Oh, I got to go pick something up from my friend's house I left there," or some stupid shit. My mom would be sitting out in front of the trap.

Jennifer's relapse was immediate. Within an hour of her release from jail, she was using again. She didn't even bother waiting until she could go by herself. Her relationship with her parents had already been significantly damaged at this stage. This wasn't her first arrest, and she stole from them long before getting caught for the first time. She knew she was on the brink of being cut off entirely. Yet, her need was so urgent that she didn't consider potential legal or personal consequences of using again.

In spite of regaining clarity while he was in jail, Dale (WM28) recalled what he believed to be the futility of the entire process. During his several periods of incarceration, he was able to reflect upon the errors that he'd made and how what he was doing was only going to lead to more trouble. Ultimately, it wouldn't matter, because as soon as he left jail, his thinking reverted, "I'm able to go to jail and then I'm able to think again. I get my thoughts back and then I'm starting to see, 'Damn, what the fuck was I doing?' Then as soon as I get out, I'm not thinking again. I'm in the moment and I'm not thinking because I find my dealer's number in my phone. I'm not thinking if I call him it's going to be this way…If I'm locked up, I can't go get it." When dope was beyond his reach, Dale was forced to recognize how he'd ended up in a jail cell and face the negative impact that heroin had on his life. He gained the ability to see multiple bad decisions into the future, piecing together how one would lead to the next, it just never lasted.

Reflecting on her past cycles of release and relapse, Rachel (WF28), had trouble comprehending how she could have been so accepting of the risk her actions invited. Periods of withdrawals and incapacitation that had only just concluded faded into the background as soon as she had her freedom. Knowing that she had done the same thing over and over evoked feelings of befuddlement,

> It gets crazy to me the situations I put myself through, not even realizing how dangerous it was. Now I'm thinking you [herself] could have just done some real major time. You just got placed under arrest and then the second night you're released you want to go fucking get high again? It was fine to me at the time. It made all the sense then…you've seen what just happened when you was trying to get drugs, but yet you're doing again. You're literally the definition of insane.

While likely not involving true psychosis, the repetition of the same harmful cycle certainly fits in a colloquial sense. The fascinating aspect of her repetition was that, in those moments, what she was doing made perfect sense. Her brain craved dope and her body was going to do whatever necessary to oblige, as if she had no memory of the consequences that had immediately preceded.

The length of time that a person spent locked up didn't change much either (Mitchell et al. 2017; Perry et al. 2015). Prior to getting arrested, Henry (WM30) had been stealing for months. He got quite good at it, doing it almost daily without getting caught. Eventually, his luck ran out, "I was stealing from Walmart. I did 18 months on that one. It was attempted robbery because I told the dude don't put his hands on me, a threat. That was back when everyone was stealing from Walmart. Went to prison, got out. Got right back to it, like I didn't skip a beat, right back to using and everything. Soon as I got out of the half-way house." After a year-and-a-half of incarceration, Henry knew he was going to go get dope. In fact, he'd started using oxys his last couple weeks in the halfway house, undoing the first 17 months throughout which he made plans for a better future.

Consequences simply did not matter for addicts determined to get out and use. A rapidly mounting criminal record could not have been less important. By this stage, their respective situations often best aligned with Sherman et al.'s (1992) conditional hypothesis, predicting that sanctions will fail to affect an individual that does not identify with attachments to conventional society. The experience of incarceration and withdrawals was miserable, sure, but the severity of a sentence only mattered in the sense that it was going to prolong his period of sobriety. The negative credential the arrest and punishment represented was irrelevant. In fact, in one example, Kathy (WF44) described how she wouldn't have minded being locked up if she had the means to avoid withdrawals, "My criminal record was getting worse…It only mattered to me in so far that I knew the penalties would be worse and I would be sick more. I truly did not care. I just didn't want to be in jail because I couldn't get high. *I'd be perfectly fine if I had gone to jail and they gave me drugs.* I just want to get out and get well."

This Time Will Be Different: Hollow Plans for a Better Future

Can getting locked up drive an addict to want to get clean? As we saw previously, going through withdrawals alone may not deter an addict from planning to cop immediately after they get out. Still, it was not as if their minds were laser focused on getting high immediately throughout their time inside. For some, interaction with the justice system, on the surface, appeared to actually have had the desired transformative effect. Incarceration gave them the moment of clarity that they needed– it was time to change. Many began to make plans for when they get out, to think about how they would do things differently this time. Withdrawing in jail was awful, getting arrested again only further alienated their friends and families, and most of all, they never wanted to find themselves in same position ever again. Unfortunately, these dreams usually remained fantasies.

Opioid addicts are well-known for their propensity to relapse– it's estimated that 91 percent will within the first year after getting clean (Smyth et al. 2010). It's an uphill climb. Even under optimal circumstances, it's far from guaranteed that putting someone through detox will have any beneficial impact on their desire to use. There's an even smaller chance that detox in a jail, absent the resources available to dedicated treatment centers, will influence lasting change.

Most addicts experienced some form of aspirational forward thinking, typically among earlier periods of incarceration, and developed some measure of buy-in to changing, the kind that was sincere. However, it proved easier to make plans than it was to have to make good on them.

They would go in wanting to use more than anything in the world, suffer through withdrawals, and then develop optimism for how things might be different when they get out, representing the positive apex of their time inside. Then, as their release date drew closer, they slowly descended into thoughts of wanting to use again, so that by the time they were released, it was as if their plans never existed. Dennis (WM27) described how this process unfolded in his mind,

> I would get right back out of jail and as much as I hated it, and as much as it killed me to be in there, I would use again…While being locked up, you get all the different thoughts as, "Okay, I'm going to change." This, that, and the third. And then right when you hit those streets again, "Boom." It's over. It's almost like you instantly forget all of the trouble you just went through. All of the pain, all of the nervousness, and the worries that you just went through in jail. You hit those streets and it's like your mind completely switches right back to drugs. In jail, you can't get stuff, so your mind is already– you're telling yourself, "Hey I can't get it. I might as well try to better myself." Start thinking different thoughts. But as soon as you hit those streets and you know that it's available, that you could get it easily and you go right back to thinking that you're going to be relaxed and stress-free, it's like, "Man, this is super hard. I thought I was going to be able to come out here and be more of a productive citizen, just because of all the hell I went through." But now that it's easily available again, it's just like you go right back to it. That addictive thinking, it's just so easy to fall right back and do that. It's ridiculous.

When he knew heroin was off the table, Dennis had the opportunity to focus on ways that he could improve his situation and the self-work that might help him not end up back in jail. At the time, having those thoughts was reassuring. He felt better about where he was– a dank, loud, open floorplan jail cell with roughly 40 other men. He could convince himself that this was the last time he'd be there. Ultimately, his situation was akin to making an empty New Year's resolution to work out every day, lose 20 pounds, and eat healthier. Problem was, actually sticking to what he aspired to was a lot harder than it sounded in his head. Each time he got out, before he knew it, he was back to using.

Raquel (BF42), who pushed into stage three when her heroin use intensified, was deep enough into her addiction to not care if she was guaranteed to be arrested. It's not that she did not want to get better– rarely is a heroin addict truly content with living at rock bottom– rather, sitting in a jail cell and fantasizing about a different future wasn't enough to make her want to quit when she knew she was about to have the chance to use again,

> When you're in there you go, "Oh, I'm never going to do it again." Yeah, it's like you make all of these promises and stuff. Who wants to be in that shit?...After a while you do feel like you want to do better. Don't get me wrong. You do want to. You know you really do want to do better. You're going to get clean. As time starts to wind down, that voice starts edging back into you. It's like a quiet one, to a louder one, and then you're getting out and all you can think about is, "I want to go get. I'm going to get it. I'm going to get it. Who am I gonna get it from?"...They call your name and as soon as you walk out, I'm already dialing the number in my head. I can't tell you the times when I came home and within 28 to 72 hours I wasn't using. I did every single time.

As her release approached, the voice in the back of her mind, the one that drove her to act on impulse and do anything in the pursuit of dope, once again grew louder. As soon as she walked out the gate, her original plans may as well have never existed.

She wasn't alone either. It was common for individuals that did time to recall having moments of clarity where they found themselves planning for a future that would never come to pass. Think back to Adam– even after he completed treatment, which afforded him greater resources than someone that receives just a jail term, all of which he enthusiastically utilized, it wasn't enough. Paul (WM34) made a plan. When he was released from jail, he wanted to do things differently. Not many actually have a concrete idea of what "different" looks like, but one certainty is that it never includes heroin. The grind his life had become was something he wanted to leave behind. Being locked up in one of the worst jails in the country made a lasting impression, but, like Raquel, his resolve started to weaken as his release date got closer, "I knew I didn't want to go back to that [addiction]. And you know, I just, I thought things were going to be different. But you know, toward the end of my sentence I'm thinking, 'I could probably get high just couple of times. Get there, hang out with my friends,' that type of thing. Because I knew once I did my time, I would be out free and clear."

Robin (W.TW27) had experienced the cycle of release and relapse before. She made plans every time she went inside. All told, her most recent drug arrest made it 15 times she'd been locked up, so she knew how the situation typically played out. While she was sober and knew she wasn't going anywhere, it was easy to embrace notions of sobriety. Deep down, Robin knew it was a long shot that things would work out. She had lost her sunny-side optimism several arrests ago,

> When you're sober you think that you're going to create this whole life, but I mean being an addict, I've created in my mind this perfect life that I'm going to have so many times and it doesn't...shit doesn't work out like that. I think that most people's problem is they don't have the support. They don't have anywhere to go. If you don't have no place to go and you go back to the same place, the same people, the same shit, same shit's going to happen.

Maybe things would have been different with a place to go, maybe not. After her first few releases, she had a place to go. Her family could only take so many thefts and dishonesties before they cut her off. The saddest part was that Robin knew herself too well. Despite wanting to do things differently and making a commitment to a new start, she relapsed within days of leaving treatment.

Having nowhere to go came up often. Many addicts had no idea what to do once they were released. It was a growing source of anxiety– they knew the date was approaching, and without a plan, they often returned to what was familiar,

> When I was in jail, I begged my mom to let me come home, and she wouldn't do it. And I just couldn't understand why she wouldn't do it. I had nowhere else to go besides the trap. So, of course I'm gonna go back and do some sort of drug, whether it was heroin or crack or whatever. I was gonna do something because the only way I would have a place to stay would be to spend money there. If they would have let me come home at that time, I probably would not have gone back to using, I probably would have stayed sober and been okay.

Holly (WF42), like Robin, had done too much damage to her family for them to want to welcome her into their home again. While she was locked up, Holly figured they would let her stay there, even if just for a few days. When that fell through, she had no back-up. It's hard to say whether she would have stayed clean, but in her mind, not having a roof over her head after she got out of jail sealed her fate.

Like Its Own Little City: Being Locked Up Isn't So Bad

A key component of specific deterrence is that an individual's direct experience with punishment will have discourage future offending (Anwar and Loughran 2011; Matsueda et al. 2006; Pogarsky and Piquero 2003). An implicit component of that equation is that being incarcerated will be miserable. Problematically, for a surprising number of addicts, incarceration was something that they feared only up until the point when they were first incarcerated. It was nothing like what they'd seen on tv or in movies. Inmates weren't getting their throats cut and people weren't being sexually assaulted left and right. The image of incarceration that they once feared, even if it wasn't enough to stop them from committing crimes to fund their addictions in the first place, no longer carried the same threat that it used to when it was a nebulous, abstract idea.

Amanda (WF30) started using percs when her stepdad introduced her to snorting them. Later on, she and the father of her first child were making Florida trips and each quickly got up to using 20 or so 30s a day. Florida dried up and she couldn't find the pills on the street for long. She made the transition to heroin and with that came crime. After she was caught selling by a sting operation, she received several felony charges, including aggravated robbery, robbery, and drug trafficking. She was lucky and was only sentenced to roughly two years in jail, a transitionary facility, and was granted parole. Though, she wasn't ready to stop using and relapsed shortly after her release. After a series of several parole violations and 60-day jail terms, the entire process became normal for Amanda,

> I wasn't scared of jail anymore. I was always thinking like, "Well, I did the big amount of time. It's just a PV (parole violation). I can do 60 days." Stupid, but, that's how I thought. I just knew that the judge...well, I thought I knew. I was like, "Well, he knows I need treatment, he's not gonna send me to prison." I'm not catching no more charges. I'm not doing things that may be soliciting, but it's a misdemeanor, you know what I mean? And they usually wanna get solicitors help. That's how I justified it, like, "Well, you're not gonna send me to prison. I'm an addict, I need help."

If anything, she had enough contact with the system to recognize that, being an addict, they weren't going to throw the book at her. She kept getting sent to treatment, getting out, relapsing, and repeating the process. It was part of the routine and none of it made her think about getting clean. She had to intermittently along the way– she couldn't avoid it when the courts sent her to treatment– but it never stuck until several years later when she became fed up with the lifestyle and decided on her own that she wanted to get help.

The circumstances surrounding Donte's (BF40) arrests were different, even if the end result was the same. He grew up in the city's worst neighborhood and never had the desire to leave. He knew everyone and everyone knew him– just how he wanted it. Part of growing up in his neighborhood meant he was always around drugs, even at a young age. He saw the nice things that the dope boys had and started selling as soon as he could. When he got a little older, he and his associates started selling percs. They were easy to get and there was a heavy market for them. Eventually, curiosity got the best of him. He developed an addiction quickly, initiating a long, circuitous path featuring several periods of incarceration, one of which was a several-year prison term. After that experience, his anxiety levels surrounding the commission of crime decreased considerably. When the sickness would set in, it drove him to take large risks. He knew what the consequences might be, but after serving that prison term, getting caught for dope-related thefts wasn't a problem at all,

> The fatigue was a little bit more extreme…you got the shits and you're like, "Damn, you can't hold nothing in." Felt clammy. It got extremely real…some of the risks you take, you just don't…I'm going to do what I've got to do, whatever it takes. Like one time I went up in a dollar store. I loaded the carts up and pushed them right up out of there like it was legal. Got $300-400 and I probably took about thousand dollars' worth of shit. I didn't care…ain't nobody worry about getting caught. Hell, we're getting caught. That's a temporary stay. What they going to do? Lock you up a few days? Petty theft, larceny… you're not worried about none of that shit at the time. Fucking 90 days, that ain't shit. I had done years. I don't worry about no 90 days. That ain't nothing.

Donte expected to get caught. When it happened, he would go do the time. He knew what to expect when he got there and having to stay for a few weeks or even months didn't bother him, certainly not enough to make him want to get clean.

Counterintuitively, the same pattern applied to others as well. Lengthier prison sentences did as much as abbreviated jail terms to discourage use. Addicts adapted quickly and settled into the repetition of daily life in prison. Anyone familiar with offenders' incarceration preferences knows that an inmate would choose to serve time in prison over jail, all things being equal. Jail is a chaotic place. Constant turnover, belligerent, inebriated, or unstable individuals– all of it breeds unpredictability. It becomes significantly more difficult to establish a sense of the environment, to get a lay of the land. Prison was attractive because it offered stability. People are not coming and going by the day, if someone had been high when they got arrested, they'd be clean before they got there. In prison, there's a routine and many take comfort in it.

Robin (W.TW27), who earlier described how her several incarcerations had not meaningfully altered her use, had a similar experience when she was sent to prison for the first time for a series of heroin-fueled robberies,

> I've been to jail so many times. I've been to every prison there is, pretty much, in Ohio. Once you've been to jail, once you've been to prison, what can somebody do to you? You know what I mean? You get to that point where you're like, "I'm not scared." Once you've passed the point where you're not scared…I would just get in the mind frame of I had to go back then. Now, if you told me I had to do six to seven years, I'd be on your fucking feet, crying, begging you not to send me back. But then, I didn't care. I would go to prison, get a boyfriend, get some money together, start snorting suboxone again, and go back down the same path. So no, it wouldn't bother me. Being in prison, it's like a whole different world.

> Being inside of them gates, them fences, it's like its own little city inside of the
> fence, and it goes fast. It does. My six years went fast.

Once she had gone to prison, there was nothing left that she feared. It wasn't her first choice, by any means, but it was doable. She wanted to use when she was free do so and she had a plan to keep using even if she was sent to prison. Either way, opioids weren't going away, and no one could tell her differently.

John (WM36) had never been to prison before. When he was charged, he was petrified of going. He'd been in and out of jail a few times, but his addiction made each one a temporary obstacle to soon be forgotten. Prison was different. He was about to do several years for opioid-related crimes, and he had no idea what to expect. Though, after a couple weeks, he realized something unexpected– it wasn't that bad,

> After I went to prison the first time, I wasn't scared to go back. You know what
> I'm saying? Like, it's not that bad. I didn't want to go back, but I wasn't scared of
> it like I was before the first time. I was scared to death of prison. I had fun the
> whole time, you know? It's not that bad. It never scared me or deterred me from
> doing anything else…you see shit from the movies and whatnot, and you think it's
> all crazy, and it's not. So, after that, I just wasn't scared to go back to jail or
> anything. Prison's like just being in a small, little city with a fence around it, you
> know?

He didn't want to go back, but if he had to? Okay. That might be the cost of getting high. He wasn't ready to quit using and now that he knew that what was supposed to be the biggest deterrent he could face wasn't anything to be afraid of, he did whatever he wanted. In a paradoxical sense, prison time was actually liberating.

Although incarceration did not have a lasting effect, and the act of being incarcerated was more tolerable than many expected after withdrawals stopped, there are other ways that the justice system can hope to keep addicts on the straight-and-narrow. Probation and/or parole offer another avenue of less restrictive supervision that could conceivably assist the desistance process. Being in the community will permit an addict to have greater access to treatment-related resources that are likely unavailable in the context of a jail or prison. Ideally, an addict can get clean in jail, be placed on community supervision, seek treatment, and be held accountable by frequent drug tests, but ideal circumstances and opioids are like oil and water.

It didn't matter if someone was on probation or parole. Using opioids was a greater imperative. It became a game of chance. In the mind of an addict, if they had you come in to drop on a Thursday, odds were they wouldn't have you come in on Friday, meaning that if they got high that night, it would likely be out of your system by Monday. Trying to reason out gaps where it was "safe" to use was a fool's errand. Probation/parole offices purposefully vary their drop requests to specifically address this issue, but, as we've seen, an addict's version of risk assessment and avoidance is suspect at best.

When Jacob (WM39) was released from jail, his arrangements were fairly standard– probation, a PO, and drug screens. He had other plans. Jacob wasn't ready to give up heroin. In his mind, he could have the best of both worlds if he was clever enough,

> I got out. I was put on probation. And then I started using again right away. I had to take drug tests. So, I was trying to go in between drug tests. That's where I started feeling iffy about it. I had dropped dirty a couple times. And that obviously then meant I thought I may get arrested because of my use. Which ultimately happened, which is why I'm here now...I thought that I could do in-

between and get away with it and thought I had a little schedule figured out, as far as what days could I use. And obviously, I could definitely use on a Friday because they don't drug test me again, earliest possible time would be Monday, so I could definitely use Friday. That limited my amounts or the way that I was doing it. But then at some point in time I just decided to say, "Fuck it, I don't care" and used. Because I'm an asshole like that.

Now sober, Jacob could look back on what he thought was a well-engineered plan and laugh, but at the time, he truly believed it would work. Opioid addiction, fundamentally, is a question of impulse control. Consequently, it's dubious to think that someone in active heroin addiction would be capable of instituting and adhering to concrete rules governing their usage, e.g., only using on certain days of the week or under specific conditions. Eventually, he could no longer tame his addiction and gave in, ignoring the boundaries he had set for himself. Using was simply a higher priority.

In similar situations, frequent drops, and the implementation of strategic plans to use, led to concentrated increases in opioid use. For example, Nancy (WF41) was aware of the risk that using carried while she was on paper, so when she made the decision to use, she was going to make it count, "I feel like when I did use, when I have a warrant or I'm on probation and I wasn't in treatment, and I use knowing that I'm going to drop dirty, I might as well make it worth my while. You know what I mean? Go big or go home. I'm not going to jail over a dime when I might as well just go and get $60 or so wanting to go to jail. That's what we say." When the goal of punishing addicts is to help them get clean, it's problematic if they OD and die. In Nancy's case, there were several instances where she was locked up, forced to get clean, and it would last a few weeks. At release, it may have been months since she used last. In that time, her tolerance was likely to have decreased, perhaps significantly. Combined with a "go big or go home" mentality created by a perceived window to use, the probability of her overdoing it is significantly higher than if she administered the same dosage in the midst of active addiction months prior.

Tim (WM33) sold drugs for several years before he became an opioid addict. Ironically, it was probation that sent him into heroin addiction. He'd tried opioids before, but at the time of his first arrest, Tim had a massive marijuana habit. He would smoke all day, every day, putting him at odds with his new requirement to drop several times a week since it stays in your system for weeks. He suffered from anxiety and was adamantly opposed to taking anti-depressants, so he decided to self-medicate with opioids instead,

> I knew opiates were out of your system quick, and I was already comfortable with the needle…I managed to use heroin for like 10 months out of my 12 months that I was supposed to be on probation, and never dropped dirty once. They had it set where every, whatever day it was. So, I gave myself like two-and-a-half to three-and-a-half days every single time, and I'd go through the sickness. For a while, I still had that willpower and that ability to, you know, those couple of days. Then as my addiction progressed over the years, I couldn't do that anymore, you know? The foundation blocks were taken out and it just weakened and weakened and weakened, and my willpower just went to shit.

Much like Jacob, Tim couldn't force himself to follow his self-imposed guidelines. Tim got lucky, or at least he thought he did. Most POs know better than to stick to a set drop schedule, but what he thought was a gift was a curse. In that ten-month period, Tim went from snorting a few perc 30s here and there to becoming a full-on, high volume IV heroin addict.

By the time of Paul's (WM34) first arrest, he had already graduated to shooting heroin. He was charged with a felony, but received a future indictment, meaning he didn't have to go to jail straight away. He spent a day or two there while they processed him out, but that was all.

Instead, they put him on paper, letting him go while the courts decided what to do with him, "Being on paper, it didn't keep me from using it. It made me worry more, but it didn't ultimately stop me. Once I got caught and got a future [indictment] in this county, I really started thinking like, 'Man, this could come back. I could be doing this all over again.' You know? But at this time, I'd already been caught for it, so it wasn't a major deterrent, no." That first day in jail was a wake-up call. As soon as he was out, he immediately started dwelling on what could happen to him if he screwed up while he was free, waiting on his indictment to come back. He couldn't imagine having to do serious time and the prospect of possibly going to prison for years scared him, knowing what it would mean for his addiction. Being an addict, Paul's response to stress was to use, effectively obscuring and erasing any concerns about future time behind bars.

Playing the Law

An important component of the demystification of incarceration was the increased familiarity with what certain crimes' punishments carried in actuality. An addict knows they're going to get caught at some point. If they've fully committed to their addiction, it's nearly an inevitability. Interestingly, how they got caught was a focus for several addicts. If they've used long enough, an addict becomes a master manipulator. Bilking friends and family from whatever money they can pry away under false pretenses or finessing doctors for scripts they never needed gave them ample practice. Although the majority were not actively trying to avoid arrest, there were ways they knew they could shield themselves of full culpability. Many knew that if there was sufficient evidence indicating that they were an addict, like being arrested with paraphernalia or drugs, there was a greater chance that they could leverage their addiction to receive a more lenient sentence.

Max (WM34) knew that he was going to get arrested sooner or later, but it didn't scare him. What made him unafraid was knowing that he was a complete mess. Take one look at him at the peak of his addiction and all you could possibly see is a strung-out train wreck of a person. By the time he started compiling multiple arrests in the span of a few weeks, he was setting the foundation to be perceived as a troubled drug addict in need of aid, "It was more okay. If I get caught selling this, I'm going to do a lot more time. But if they catch me and I've only got a small amount on me that I'm using and I've got my utensils, they're going to label me as an addict and I'm not going to get as much time." When he picked up selling to help subsidize his heroin habit, Max knew the risks. He had no prior arrests and was once a successful business owner, already giving him an advantage in the eyes of the court. If he kept selling, the safest way to do it was to only have a small amount on him at any given time. Combined with his injection kit, a judge with half of a heart is going to see an individual in the throes of addiction, assuming the heroin on him was for personal use, rather than someone else.

Patrick (WM44) had been in trouble a few times before his first opioid arrest, but he never spent more than a month in jail for any of it. It was only after he became an addict that his rap sheet started to grow. Over time, he recognized that being arrested without evidence that he was an addict was actually hurting him,

> I don't give a shit if I got caught because I would rather get caught with paraphernalia or drugs so they could help me. Because I never got help until they caught me with it on me. And then they gave me a future [indictment] that I never got. They never brought it back up, but ever since that charge in 2012, I get the drug and alcohol judges. You know it's like, they know you're a fucking drug addict, so they try to help even if I don't know it. You know? They're trying to help me. This is my fourth parole violation, man. I begged them to just let me do

> my jail time, but that's easy way because I could do that and not have no
> probation, and just get fucked up. You know?

With a certain sense of impunity, Patrick was even less afraid of getting arrested. He felt as

though he was free to do as he needed, knowing that if he were to be arrested in the middle of

committing a crime to fund his addiction, it was likely that he would be able to get help. In his

mind, it was a win-win; get high now and get help eventually if it was meant to be.

When an addict was arrested and it was clear that they were using, as it was with both

Max and Patrick, they were often given the choice to participate in drug court. In the immediate

stages, the opportunity to have a felony downgraded to a misdemeanor by completing the

program didn't factor into the decision to accept the deal or not. Instead, the choice to enter into

drug court was simple, but not for the reason that was intended. If they agreed to the terms, they

would be released as soon as the same day. For an addict in the first 48 hours of withdrawals, a

get-out-of-jail-free card, no matter the future costs or commitments, was an opportunity that they

could not refuse.

Deep into heroin use, Amy (WF31) saw drug court as a lifeline. In the beginning, it was

an avenue to get out and keep using, "At first, it was a way to get out. I just wanted to get out. I

wanted to be done with jail. At first, that's what it was…Within a week [after release], I

overdosed three times." Getting arrested and experiencing the early stages of withdrawal would

have led Amy to do nearly anything to get back on the street. Being confined was a threat to her

ability to use and she overcorrected once they let her go. Having felt the threat that getting

locked up posed to her ability to stay well, she dove into her habit with a vengeance. She was

afraid of being taken back to jail again, and her way of coping with the anxiety surrounding the

potential inability to use was to use more.

Joseph (WM30) made the same decision. It was almost reflexive, a characteristic common to addicts (Biernacki et al. 2018; MacKillop et al. 2011; Redish, Jensen, and Johnson 2008). The offer to get out immediately was a dream come true. Though, it became a burden after the fact, given the rigorous demands of the program, "I messed up when I came down to the plea deal. I haven't been sentenced in the drug program, but I almost want to go see how many days I can serve in jail and be done with it instead. I did it because I got out of jail, pretty much. Get released on a OR (own recognizance). I didn't know it would be anything like this. I heard "drug court," and was like, 'Hell, yeah. Get released today? Got to do drug court? Okay. Let me go.'"

Jennifer (WF31) also had the same proposition given to her, albeit under messier circumstances,

> I got charged with a bunch of drug shit, all the paraphernalia, all types of charges. I don't even know what, because from joining drug court, I think that they're dropping my charges lower. The day after I got to jail, I was supposed to go to court, I was dope sick. Extremely dope sick. I was in the back of the inner chambers chained to a wall because I have multiple felonies…I threw up all over myself so I couldn't go to court. So, they brought me back downstairs. I had to wait a whole 'nother seven days before I could go to court. By then I was feeling better…The lawyer approached me in the jail cell and said, "Hey, is this something you're willing to do?" I said, "Will I get out of jail today?" She said, "Yeah." I said, "Sign me up." And guess what I did when I got out? I got high, and I got high, and I kept getting high, and I kept getting high.

If she'd been able to keep her stomach in check, Jennifer would have been able to get out and keep using as much as she wanted within 36 hours of being picked up. Despite the delay, when presented with the same opportunity, she wasn't going to let it pass her by. It wasn't because she

wanted help, but because she didn't want to be sick any longer.

PART III. Sick and Tired of Being Sick and Tired: Cognitive Change and Getting Clean

If there's no deterring addicts, and locking them up is unlikely to make a dent in their desire to use, then what can be done? What, if anything, can policy realistically hope to achieve? It's a difficult, yet essential question. The answer is as elusive, if not more so, than any other criminal justice issue. The complex interplay between physical dependency, neurological change, emotional instability, and individual factors and circumstances introduces variability that is difficult to consistently account for.

Getting clean wasn't a logical process. The cliché "hitting bottom" is as close of a descriptor as there is for the point where everything "clicks." In reality, it's more complicated than that. For the justice-involved, this is especially true. While an individual might have the desire to change, as we saw, that can be derailed by something as ostensibly benign as being released from jail. An addict's sobriety is fragile. There are no one-size-fits-all progressions through addiction that can predict the efficacy of arrests or incarcerations, but, for most addicts, justice contact didn't matter much. Instead, it was the cumulative influence of several concurrent personal factors that proved to be the strongest influences in the development of a wholehearted commitment to getting sober. In this section, I delve deeper into these influences, discussing the roles that burnout, strained relationships, abject poverty, intense feelings of hopelessness, and ominous futures played in motivating change, exploring how they conform with influential criminological theories of cognitive change, personal identity, and criminal involvement.

Chapter 6. Cognitive Change and Desistance from Crime

The Theory of Cognitive Change and Offending

At a certain point, an offender that desists from crime will make the determination that doing crime is no longer compatible with their view of themselves, nor their personal desires. The specifics and circumstances surrounding this evolution are somewhat contested, but the underlying focus remains on the recognition of an incongruence between reality and desire, sparking meaningful change. Giordano and colleagues' (2002) were one of the most visible works of an emerging focus on the primacy of personal change in the desistance process. The authors built off of Sampson and Laub's (1993) work on turning points, which examined the factors that contributed to the desistance process among a sample of delinquent, young white males (Glueck and Glueck 1950). The pair had concluded that, while their sample was still likely to continue to offend in the future, there were detectable patterns that predicted greater probability of desistance. Specifically, individuals who had greater levels of pro-social bonds, such as marriage or employment, were more likely to reduce future offending than those that did not. The effects did not occur immediately; rather, it took time for prosocial bonds to amass and to also impact an offender meaningfully. Since the authors' publication, others have rigorously examined the theory through additional empirical work, with many studies supporting for Sampson and Laub's conclusions (Horney, Osgood, and Marshall 1995; King, Massoglia, and Macmillan 2007; Uggen 2000).

However, Giordano et al. (2002), among others, raised concerns regarding the thoroughness of the theory, especially with regard to the generalizability of the marriage effect across both male and female offenders as well as adolescent offenders (Graham and Bowling 1995; Horwitz and White 1987). From this position, the Giordano et al. sought to amend the theory through the incorporation of symbolic interactionist theory in the effort to better account for individual-level, reflexive processes (Dietz and Burns 1992; Giddens 1984).

On a fundamental level, moving away from familiar, habitual action requires a "cognitive shift," in order for the introduction of a pro-social bond to affect meaningful change. A would-be ex-offender cannot transition away from a life of crime unless they are first open to do so. Without a willingness to consider change, punishment or public derision may only seek to further alienate an individual, pushing them further into criminal thinking or socially deviant subculture (Becker 1963; Braithwaite 1989; Chiricos et al. 2007). This primary step is especially relevant in the study of drug users. As shown in the previous chapter, punishment alone did little to dissuade opioid users from pursuing their addictions. In keeping with other work that has concluded that drug addicts fare better once they have developed an openness to change (Bachman et al. 2016; Kay and Monaghan 2019; Rowlands, Youngs, and Canter 2020), it may be the case here as well that opioid users must first demonstrate a willingness to commit to a new lifestyle before opioid cessation.

By accounting for internal thought processes prior to a response to a pro-social opportunity, Giordano et al. (2002) introduced a novel wrinkle that expanded control theory, perhaps helping to explain variability in offenders' response to opportunities to change. For the authors, these opportunities represented potential "hooks for change." If an individual was open to the notion of changing their behavior, exposure to an avenue to do so then had the potential to act as a catalyst for a new way of living. The process, again, did not happen immediately, nor was an openness to change sufficient on its own. Rather, continued exposure, or the exposure to several hooks, was an important part of the process. Throughout, the authors maintained that an offender may begin to see the merits of changing as time passed. Behaviors that they had previously found unappealing began to appear increasingly enticing, such as learning a trade, pursuing an education, or committing to a "respectable" relationship.

When an offender began to develop meaningful cognitive connections with a given opportunity (e.g., employment), they initiated a reflexive process of critically examining the future. As an individual's connections strengthened, they increasingly recognized the existence of an alternative path. They no longer felt that they had only one possible life ahead of them. In a sense, their eyes began to open to the possibilities that might await them if they were able to leave behind the old version of themselves. By envisioning a "replacement self," an offender developed an identity-in-waiting that could ultimately be seen as capable of overwriting who they used to be.

In many instances, addicts do not have lives full of positive experiences that pre-dated addiction. In fact, many had dealt with addiction issues since their teenage years. When faced with this reality, the recognition of an alternative, less-trying way of living might be an epiphany of sorts. Sure, they were aware of what a "normal" life would have looked like, but the thought that it could belong to them was a foreign concept. Once the opportunity presents itself that it was not only possible, but also attainable, changing increasingly feels realistic.

The last stage in Giordano et al.'s (2002) conceptual process is the "transformation." By this time, an individual has desisted from crime. Their lives have changed such that they have developed solid bonds rooted in conventional ways of living. In order to mark the completion of the process, an individual must see deviant behaviors, which were previously viewed as acceptable or even desirable, as negative. The thought of behaving as they previously had in the past, such as using opioids, becomes something that they would not advocate, and certainly would not revisit themselves, coming full-circle.

While there is heavy overlap between Paternoster and Bushway (2009) and Giordano et al. (2002), the former sought to amend the latter in ways that are important for consideration in this study. As discussed, Giordano et al. (2002) heavily stress the role of social processes. Namely, they hold that individuals must have consistent hooks for change that present the opportunity to modify behavior as part of their desistance process. Paternoster and Bushway (2009) take a slightly different approach, maintaining that behavioral alteration has less to do with social context as it does with internal desire. Whereas Giordano et al. (2002) would argue that the first step in the desistance process is an openness to change, Paternoster and Bushway (2009) take the position that this step must be more resolute. Prior to connecting to and developing bonds with conventional sources, offenders must first make a conscious, personal choice to commit to forming a new identity; only then are they able to reap the full extent of the rewards of pro-social ties. Ultimately, for Paternoster and Bushway (2009), the desistance process boils down to a resolute decision to no longer engage in crime.

While the underlying mechanism is simple, its practical execution is unpredictable and messy. Individuals introduce considerable variability regarding their assessments of hooks for change and their respective timelines for fully desisting. In Paternoster and Bushway's (2009) view, the desistance process is not boiled down to easily identifiable, acute opportunities; rather, "desistance from crime involves important changes in a person's identity, tastes, values, and preferences" (p. 1108-09). To make a full break, an individual must change their identity by moving away from their view of themselves as someone that does crime.

158

Preceding the decision-making process, an offender must, in some fashion, amass experiences that make them question the path that they are on. When negative events and feelings accumulate, an offender may project the circumstances of a given moment into the future. Specifically, if they are fully dissatisfied with the present, they must contemplate whether there is any reason to think that the future will be different unless they change their behavior. When an offender encounters this "feared self," the authors would argue that it will serve as the impetus for the development and commitment to better "future self," characterized by altered behaviors. Consequently, individuals will then begin to embrace opportunities to form beneficial bonds in order to actualize their desired future identity.

Identity-based Change and Recovery

Research with specificity to desistance from drug use and addiction, rather than crime in an overarching sense, shares many of the same underlying identity change-related suppositions. The dominant perspectives on addiction recovery typically fall into one of two general theories. On one hand, some believe that maintaining sobriety is an ongoing process that is intimately tied to the attainment of an elevated quality of life that stems from feelings of empowerment and self-determination (De Maeyer et al. 2011; De Maeyer, Vanderplasschen, and Broekaert 2009). A prominent example of this school of thought is the well-known Narcotics Anonymous (NA) program, which treats addiction as a chronic condition requiring methodical, continuous attention (Kay and Monaghan 2019). This perspective is compatible with both Giordano et al. (2002), as well as Maruna (2001), who still consider internal desire important, but regard social context as more central to the desistance process.

On the other, the Therapeutic Communities model (De Leon 2000) holds that addiction is an affliction that can be conquered. In that sense, an individual that completes programming and develops an internal commitment to "right living" transforms themselves into former addicts, no longer requiring ongoing treatment or addiction-related social support, such as in the former view. Given the considerable separation between the two perspectives' conceptions of the personal actions necessary to ensure recovery, there is important disagreement regarding the most effective approach to treatment. Similar to Paternoster and Bushway's (2009) thoughts regarding desistance from crime, the Therapeutic Communities model maintains that identity change is a central component of the recovery process (Biernacki 1986), arguing that a new identity grounded in sober living must supplant an addict's sense of self formed during active addiction. A conscious break with a prior reality is necessary in order to begin a new, sober chapter, leaving behind what some have called the "spoiled self" (McIntosh and McKeageny 2002). In this sense, maintaining sobriety becomes less about social context or opportunities for change, such as those emphasized in Giordano et al. (2002), and instead asserts that the most central influence in recovery will come from within.

Chapter 7. Finding The Breaking Point: The Process of Deciding to Quit

No singular factor made an addict get clean. Instead, it was the accumulation of several concurrent experiences, the sum of which formed a critical mass whereby an addict finally reached a breaking point. In their minds, they were finally done using; this time it was the *real* thing. Getting to this point was often a long, arduous path filled with negative events that a non-drug user would likely expect to dissuade someone from continuing to use long before that was actually the case. As we saw in my participants' responses to deterrence, traditional conceptions of logic do not apply. The relentless pursuit of a singular goal cultivates an obliviousness to normative behavioral expectations, an immunity to purportedly effective consequences, and an indifference to external influence, even when coming from loved ones. Simply put, there was no way to make an addict achieve lasting sobriety unless they had reached a point in their trajectory characterized by complete and utter exhaustion, facilitating critical self-reflection, the recognition of a feared self, and the cultivation of an organic desire to quit. Then, and only then, were they ready to embrace the struggle of getting clean.

Everyone's bottom is different. Regardless of circumstance, gender, or socioeconomic status, the only commonality across my sample was that reaching a true, personal bottom was an essential component of the decision to get clean. As we saw, the probability of success is likely to be quite low when punishment is the primary means of facilitating desistance. If an addict stops using for any reason other than personal desire, they will fail. Frequently, addicts cited personal disappointment and disbelief of their circumstances, suicidal ideation, abject poverty, the alienation of friends and family, exhaustion, and advanced age as some of the most recognizable characteristics of what their bottom looked like. Here, I'll unpack these overlapping and interwoven themes, taking a deeper look at addicts' commentary on the inflection point that saw them embrace personal progressions to sobriety. First, I'll begin by examining variability in the extent of addicts' downward progressions as well as their collective recognition of the importance of hitting bottom as an antecedent of transitioning to sobriety and developing a future self (Paternoster and Bushway 2009).

The Importance of Hitting Bottom and the Ability to Keep Digging

There was no possibility of getting clean without first hitting bottom. Often, as conditions worsened, fledgling addicts began to realize that a "bottom" was nothing like they thought it would be. Compared to pre-addiction times, the notion of what constituted an "end of the world" event devolved into circumstances that were once unimaginable. Days where considering missing an electrical bill payment as a crisis of conscience transformed into significantly darker problems. In that sense, addicts often experienced a series of increasingly dire bottoms as their addictions progressed. Leslie (WF33) described how this process unfolded during her addiction and how drugs had caused her life to change,

> I never in my life thought that my bottom in my 20s wasn't really it. It was like, being late on my car payment was my bottom before, you know what I mean? What this year has been like for me, my actual bottom bottom, it was two completely different things…literally being homeless and not knowing where I was going to stay, while being pregnant. Yeah. Would've never ever pictured that my life would be like that. It's definitely my real bottom. Lowest point.

In the course of her addiction, Leslie's changing awareness of her situation was the foundation for her turning point. The distance she felt between what constituted a problem in her prior life and her life as an addict elicited feelings of disbelief. She had fallen so far during the course of her heroin addiction that she found herself pregnant, homeless, and alone. Today, in retrospect, this was her recognition of a feared self. If she were to continue on the path of addiction, there was the potential that she could find an even deeper bottom. That was a notion that she could not entertain. Somehow, she thought, she had to leave behind her spoiled self and get back to where she once was (McIntosh and McKeageny 2002).

Amy (WF31) also experienced a series of worsening bottoms. As her heroin tolerance kept increasing, the financial demands became a devastating influence on her well-being. In addition to failing health from constant use, her series of worsening bottoms saw her systematically lose all of her possessions and drive away anyone that cared for her,

> The usage always got higher…That was my bottom and it just kept bottoming. I lost everything. I mean, I was extremely unhealthy. I wasn't eating. I was homeless. I was living in my car. I had pushed everybody away from me. I had pretty much completely lost my kids at that point. Thank God they were so young, and I was able to come back from that. But I had everything and everyone good in my life, I had pushed away. I had isolated so much. They were all gone. There was nobody to turn to anymore.

After getting clean, Amy retraced how things fell away, one by one. In the moment, she recognized things were slowly worsening, but it never fully registered. They never added up. Each event was isolated, occurring amidst the struggle of chasing dope that ensured compartmentalized thinking and a lack of meaningful reflection. She hadn't lost enough. You'd imagine it's hard to fail to notice going from living under a roof to living in a car, but she was incapable of properly processing the significance of it and implications of her withering resources and relationships, facilitating an incremental descent into despair. It was only after she was finally able to take stock of the accumulation of the damage that she wanted sobriety.

The process was always clearer in hindsight. In the moment, the identification of the laundry list of problems was difficult. Hitting bottom was more of an overwhelming feeling, the fine details of which were left to be unpacked at a later date. As both women mentioned, perceptions regarding what constituted a bottom was capable of changing over time, often driven by the comparison of pre-addiction life to current circumstances. Just when they thought their lives were as bad as they could get, they got worse.

Amanda (WF30) had a similar experience. Without having lost everything, she was able to cling to remnants of the past, regardless of any ongoing problems. Although each successive bottom caused her more distress than the last, they did not cause her *enough* distress to change her behavior. Reaching her final bottom required losing it all,

> One time that I thought was the bottom was probably when I was on life support. I really thought like, "Damn, this is it. You don't ever wanna do this again. You don't wanna go through this again." But it wasn't it...It just...It wasn't. I had so much more to lose. I still had things to lose...It's kind of like you get that little bit of clean time, and the devil's like waiting on you to come out the door so he can jump on your ass. You know what I mean? He's just waiting.
>
> I finally want it. This is what I want. I came to treatment on my own. I want it now. I wanna live. I wanna be sober. I wanna get help. I hit rock bottom. I finally realized that you can't do drugs and do anything else. If you do drugs, everything you do is gonna be about that drug or related to it in some type of way…I just was done. I don't wanna do that anymore, I don't wanna suffer anymore, 'cause it eventually gets to the point where the drugs don't mask it. You're just fucking miserable. I guess that's really the difference… I was walking the streets, tricking, and it just was rough. It was so rough. Just a fucked-up situation. You don't really have nowhere to stay. You don't have things. Before, I had all these things. When it comes down to it, nobody wants you around, you know what I mean?

In treatment, it's called "HALT," you're Hungry, Angry, Lonely and Tired, and that pretty much sums it up. That's when you hit your rock bottom. You're hungry because you don't eat, you spend all your money on drugs, you're angry 'cause you just spent all your damn money on your drugs, and you're lonely because nobody wants to fucking be around somebody like that, and then you're tired because you don't fucking sleep, or you're just tired. It's just isn't fun anymore. There's nothing...It's more of just...You're just chasing drugs all day long, doing them, and not even really getting high. It's just miserable, just do it repetitive…If you haven't hit rock bottom yet, in your mind you still think, "Oh, well, I can do it again, just this time I'm gonna control it."

Amanda had to burn through every resource she had before she could commit to recovery. Nearly dying couldn't make her stop; she still had more to lose. The allure of getting high again was too strong. With each relapse, she convinced herself that it would be different, that she could control it now that she knew why it got bad the times before. Her attempts at quitting never worked because her heart wasn't in it. In the absence of full commitment, opportunities to change were no match for the "devil" that would inevitably exploit any shred of a desire she had to keep using.

In addition to personal experiences, addicts recognized the importance of hitting bottom through their relationships with other addicts. John (WM36) used for several years before getting clean. All-told, it took him roughly 15 years to finally hit his bottom. His tolerance for misery was considerably higher than many acquaintances', driven by a fierce resistance to change. On a more general level, though, he spoke about the relativity of the process and how others' thinking differed from his own,

They [addicts] just got to be fucked up long enough. They got to be at the bottom, but people's bottoms are different, you know? Some people's bottoms are gonna be as a millionaire and just be emotionally beat up, or another person's bottom is living on the fucking streets. They just have to hit their bottom. That's the only way a person's going to want to change. And it could be even seeing somebody like that, you know? Like, "Damn, I see that motherfucker sleeping in that cardboard box, that's a bottom, I don't want to be there." They got to hit bottom…They just have to reach that point in their life where they don't want to be down further than what they already are.

As Paternoster and Bushway (2009) would expect, it took John developing a feared self before he could get clean, but that came years later. He'd seen the same thing happen with others. In their cases, the time when that happened varied. For someone like John, it took a lot more than seeing someone living in a cardboard box, but he was cognizant of the fact that a feared self can also be influenced by others' addictions. We'll discuss his progression in more detail later on, but his descent halted due to a recognition of the duration of his addiction and what persisting in addiction would likely produce.

Joel's (WM35) final bottom was ultimately on the less severe end of the spectrum. Through his many years spent in addiction, he was exposed to a great deal of other addicts' experiences, which he often compared with his own, "Some people's bottoms are a lot lower than others. I mean, I would never have dreamed of doing what I did then, now that I'm sober...I was at a point where I was starving to death, eating food out of trashcans, and digging out of trashcans. I had a roof over my head, but it wasn't mine. Doing whatever it takes, having thoughts of almost murdering people to get $20 to stay well for a few hours. I'd never done that before [using]." Joel's personal bottom was relatively less dire than someone like Leslie, Amy, or Amanda. He never ended up living on the streets, but that didn't mean his bottom was less impactful. Rather, his equivalent of a breaking point was more easily reached. Throughout his struggles, although he remembered seeing others doing considerably worse circumstantially, he still recognized how far he had fallen when he was contemplating murder for drugs. For him, that was the bottom. If he could do that, he thought, who knew how far he could fall?

Dennis (WM27) provided another example of the impact of a relatively lesser bottom. With over a decade in the drug selling business, he interacted with his fair share of addicts before he became one himself. Although many acquaintances of his hit bottoms he regarded to be more severe than his own, reflecting on his experiences in addiction, he recognized that whatever a person's respective bottom was, it was essential that they found it before they could begin recovery.

> I do feel that a lot of people do have to hit rock bottom before they even want to change. Because there's only so much that you can go through, regardless of how stubborn you are, what you want to do. Drug addiction will take you to that lowest point in life…you don't have family that will support you, so you're basically starving. And then right once you get back out [of jail], then you're right back to the streets with nothing. And definitely I feel like that's rock bottom…it would take you to go through the absolute rock bottom to where you can't take it anymore, or it's getting to the point to where you're doing so bad in your life it's almost even impossible to take care of your addiction. I know people without limbs that are still out there every day fighting for their addiction, figuring out ways. So, some people it takes more, some people it takes less.

In David's mind, heroin was powerful enough that he wasn't sure it was possible to even consider change until he'd hit a bottom. It had to come first. His addiction kept blinders on him. Prior to David asking for drug court, there were times where he thought he had hit his bottom. In reality, he had further to go. He wasn't done because he hadn't suffered enough. He had more to lose. Fortunately for him, he reached that point while he still had all of his limbs.

The drive to continue to use is both complicated and exceedingly simple. In spite of the litany of awful things that resulted from heroin use on the way to a bottom, addicts loved it more than anything else in the world. An addict's ability to remain unaffected by negative experiences as their world unraveled was remarkable. Nothing demonstrated the tolerance for withstanding the toll that addiction took on their well-being as acutely as an overdose. For someone that is not an addict, a near-death experience would very likely drive them to, at minimum, strongly reconsider whatever action they took that put them in that position. An opioid addict is different. The lengths that addicts would go to in order to maintain their habit was, at times, unfathomable. It was common for an addict to have several overdoses in the course of their addiction, especially among heroin and/or fentanyl users.

The first overdose was usually the one that left a mark on the mind of an addict. It would ultimately be a temporary one, but they didn't know that at the time. In the moment, that overdose often felt like the beginning of a new era, a push to be better. Though, they soon came to find that their addiction was stronger than their ability to maintain that perspective. As time passed, sometimes in as little as a few days, the memory of the severity of the event faded. Michelle (WF28) experienced this sort of progression in the period following her first overdose,

> The first one really, really impacted me. Then what would end up happening is I would get a month clean and I'd have no tolerance and I would use, and as soon as I would start using, it'd be like, maybe four times in a week, I would overdose. And really quickly for me, it became like, "Oh, well, whatever. It just happened again; this is inconvenient." "Now 911's here," or "Whatever, I'm at the hospital again. I have to find a ride home." It just seemed inconvenient to me, like "This just happened." Sometimes I'd be disappointed, like, "Really? Did that really just

happen again?" But it really gets to a point where death isn't scary anymore. And part of me, at this point, I really OD'd a lot. And it's like, "If that's what it feels like to die, what is there to be afraid of?"

After multiple overdoses, the prospect of dying wasn't scary anymore. She became desensitized to the gravity of what was becoming habitual. In her mind, the odds were that she would come out of the overdose fine; someone would help bring her back like they had before. Even in those instances where she had a glimmer of a thought that would make her consider quitting, it was no match for the momentum her addiction had generated.

Kevin's (WM23) first overdose was a memorable, traumatic experience. His family found him lying in the garage, unresponsive. They were already aware of the extent of Kevin's drug problem; he had arrived home from rehab a few days prior. They didn't know it then, but that OD, and its proximity to him "quitting" was a portent of what was to come over the next few years,

> I've had three ODs. Didn't even fucking faze me. Did not faze me. The only time one did was because my parents found me in the garage. Because I had just gotten out of rehab, my first rehab. My parents found me. It was like 5:00 in the morning. My dad was doing CPR, chest compressions on me. And my sister and my brother were out there. So that, super visceral, graphic, graphic stage...I was like, "I swear to God, I'm done. I'm done." And I meant it too. But I was not. I wasn't done yet...Two of them [ODs], I had just gotten out of treatment and almost immediately relapsed. And then the third one was mixing benzodiazepines and opioids and I just fell out. Other than the garage one, no. I felt guilt and shame for putting my family through that. Even though I was a shell of a person, I still knew that that must have been terrible. But the other two didn't faze me. One of them, I woke up in the hospital and I was like, "Yep, it's time to go," which is crazy to think about now. I just woke up and basically tore the IV out of my arm and walked out...Didn't faze me at all. I think the gravity of the situation, I was so

wrapped up in my own bullshit, the gravity never really, like, "Oh, you literally almost just died." Like, "You have fluid in your lungs, and you're about to die" never hit me.

Kevin was sincere– he wanted to quit, and it was because of what had happened that night in the garage. It was partially because of the risk, but it was also out of concern and consideration for the impact it had on his family. He stayed clean for a time, but the strength of the memory and the determination that stemmed from it faded. When he relapsed, he knew the danger he was placing himself in. It didn't matter.

Over time, as in Kevin's case, overdoses became events that were nothing more than a mile marker. Another reference point on a journey towards individuals' respective bottoms. This was the case for Steve (WM44). His first overdose didn't do much to dissuade him from using in the long term, although it did scare him at first. After the second, it became normal for him, so much so that having more than one in the same day didn't dampen his desire to keep using,

> I'm in the grocery store bathroom. I got a boy from Detroit coming down, bringing me a bunch of dope, so I'm like, "I want to try it out before I buy anything from you." So, he gives me like half a gram of shit. He's like, "Man, just be careful with it." I go in the bathroom and I do a shot of it. I don't do much, and I wake up in the hospital. I'm like, "Son of a bitch." So, I leave. I take the IV out and I just leave. I don't sign no papers, no shit like that. Who cares? I go back to the grocery store. Guess what I find on the floor? My dope. So, I do it again. This time, I break my ankle because I'm straddled on the toilet using the back of the commode as a table, and my ankle gets wedged between the toilet and the wall. So, I break my ankle. So, I go back a third time with the broken ankle and then I OD again. Three times in the same bathroom.

Broken ankle and all, Steve decided to hobble his way back to the grocery store thinking that the third time would be the charm. The idea of shooting the very dope that nearly killed him twice earlier the same day wasn't enough to dissuade him. After the second, rather than concern for his well-being, his mind went back to the bathroom– wondering what the odds were his dope might still be in the bathroom again. The intensity of Steve's indifference to death was startling. He reached a point in his addiction where his focus on a singular goal got him stuck in a loop where touching the metaphorical hot stove had no effect. In a practical sense, think of it this way– if he wasn't deterred from using the same dope again after two near-death experiences earlier the same afternoon, is it reasonable to think that the threat of going to jail would scare him into not using?

Greg (WM29) was similarly unaffected by his accumulation of overdoses. For him, it was the transition to fentanyl that left him most vulnerable. More volatile than heroin, the margin for error when estimating how much to use at any given time was considerably smaller than with tar or China. Nevertheless, it hit harder and that was what he was after, regardless of the risk it posed,

> Eventually, pills led into heroin, and heroin led into fentanyl. When I got introduced to fentanyl, I was dying left and right. I have no tolerance to it. Like I said, I've been brought back on Narcan 11 times, and the rest of the times that I've OD'd it was on my own will coming back. I've OD'd over 20 times…as soon as I came back, I wanted more. It didn't affect me like, "Hey, this shit's killing me." It's seeking that… *It's seeking to die*. Then, when you do overdose, you don't know it's happening. You just think you're getting that rush, and then when it does happen, you're waking up with fucking Narcan or in a hospital. You don't remember nothing. All it is, is just a black light like you're asleep. That's all it is.

Every time he overdosed, he never felt like something dangerous was happening in that moment. It was death disguised as the ordinary rush he associated with IV opioid use, and he was none the wiser. Without knowing any better, he thought he was getting exactly what he signed up for.

Consequently, it becomes easier to understand how an addict becomes numb to the effects of an overdose. If the only irregularity between an OD and when he was using any ordinary Tuesday night was waking up in a hospital or to a friend holding Narcan, the gravity of the event may fail to influence his thinking.

Overdoses were also frequently accompanied by compounding medical issues, exacerbated by addicts' devotion to IV use. Not only were ODs immediate threats to their lives, but underlying medical issues associated with them also posed grave danger. Heroin's pull becomes especially evident when you consider how someone like Patrick (WM44) developed such a myopic view of his well-being, "This last time, I almost died. I OD'd three times that week. I had this abscess on the back of my head. I don't know how I got it. The motherfucker was like a softball and it was green. It was gonna get into my blood system, but I couldn't make it to the hospital because I had to get a dime [of heroin] before I could go...Me getting high was more important than if that was gonna kill me, you know what I mean? That's crazy." In spite of the danger presented by an abscess on his head that looked like an unripened orange, Patrick was set on continuing on a path that had nearly killed him several times that week. Neither overdoses nor other threats to his health could dissuade him from getting high.

Nicole (AF26) had been an IV heroin user for several months before she started to have serious complications stemming from her use. One day, she used several times but still could not shake what she assumed was dope sickness. In the process, she ended up overdosing and found herself at a hospital where they gave her surprising news,

> I could not get well, and I ended up going to the hospital because I couldn't breathe. They said I had pneumonia in both lungs. I spent three months in the hospital. They said I have congestive heart failure. I ended up getting a blood

> infection and that went to my heart…I was still underweight and everything when
> I got out, and they tell me the next time I shot dope it would kill me. Well, the
> same day I got out I shot dope in the parking lot leaving the hospital…They told
> me, "If you use again you're going to die." I had pneumonia on top of it, but I still
> used the same day they told me it would kill me.

Despite being told in no uncertain terms that she would die if she used again, Nicole couldn't

stop. She didn't want to. After three months in the hospital, it was all she wanted. She couldn't

even make it out of the parking lot of the hospital. Without using in so long, shooting posed an

even greater risk of triggering an overdose due to her reduced tolerance, but she wasn't going to

stop just because someone told her to.

Nearly everyone became desensitized to the prospect of overdosing, but it didn't mean

they weren't trying to avoid it. Even if it was still likely, there was a recognition that not having

one was beneficial. Nevertheless, they accepted the inherent risk of shooting dope. For Paul

(WM34), the key was to find that sweet spot between using less and getting high, but doing so

was difficult,

> I tried to make an effort on how much I used. I would use what some would
> consider a very, very small amount. I don't know if it's because my system was so
> fresh getting out of prison, but I mean it was like I would use almost nothing. Like
> a $10.00 bag, my mom could do three or four of, I would have to do half of that,
> and even sometimes a quarter of it…The weird thing about overdosing with
> Narcan is sometimes I didn't even know it happened. I remember one very clearly,
> I was waiting on dinner to get done. And it's like I sat up and my plate was there,
> and no one had said anything to me. I looked down and I seen a Narcan thing on
> the floor and I'm like, "Where'd that come from?" They're like, "You just
> overdosed." I had no recollection of anything happening. In fact, I was still
> looking for my shot. I know I made it. Because I didn't feel any different. That
> happened several times. I mean it's really strange… After 20-30, I was trying to

use as sparsely as possible. It's like I really didn't try to use that much anyway. So, I'm like at a quarter of a bag or you know, a quarter of a $10.00 bag, it's like I really can't do any less and not feel anything. So, it was just depending on the mixture sometimes of whether or not I'd overdose.

Buying dope in 2019 was always a gamble. Whatever Paul could get off the streets was a mystery bag. How much of it was dope? How much of it was cut? Who knew how much of it was fentanyl? He never truly knew the answer to any of those questions. The only way to find out was to shoot it and deal with the consequences later. He wasn't very good at it either. Ultimately, Paul estimated that he'd had over 15 overdoses during his active use. If not for his multifunctional partner/babysitter/Narcan-administrator, he'd probably be dead.

Overdoses could also serve a greater purpose. It was rarely the event that drove people to say "enough," but an overdose was capable of planting a seed that made them question their trajectory. It varied from person to person. Over the years, Nick (WM43) lost track of how many overdoses he had. All he knew was that it was a lot more than 10. With an estimated 70 drug arrests since the age of 12, Nick was well-accustomed to the lifestyle. Going to jail was expected, just like dying was. The past three decades were all sort of a blur, littered with memories of the most noteworthy events, including his worst overdoses. Somewhat recently, Nick had one that started him thinking that maybe, after all this time, he should give sobriety a try,

> We was driving from the North side to the South side of the city. And we had just got some dope, and my wife was driving and we was arguing about something. I shot the shot…She looked over and I was turning blue and then she pulled off on the side of the road, got me out the car, and started doing CPR on me. She called the ambulance. She said some girls pulled up and helped her, but they hit me with four Narcan and I didn't come back until I was halfway to the hospital. They had a

sheet over me in the ambulance, pronounced dead and everything. They said I just sat up. I had the sheet on my head and I'd just sit up and I'm like, "Where am I? What's going on?" They just like, "You're dead." And it felt for real.

That's the first time I thought about really getting clean. I thought seriously about getting clean because I thought I was dead. I thought I was like, I don't know where I was. I was in another dimension. I didn't know what was going on…I'm like, "Damn, I don't want to leave my family. I don't want to leave my kids and my grandkids." And my wife, she's crying in the hospital room and it just broke my heart. To realize what I'm doing to them or how I was going to leave them and how they was going to feel if I died…What I was doing to them, it was the first time I actually seen the effects and really looked at what I was doing to them. And then it broke my heart.

I still got high a couple days later. I really didn't want to, but I didn't want to be sick either. I had tried to hold out as long as I felt I could. I tried to use just a little bit so that I wouldn't be sick. But then after I used heroin, it gets in the back of my addicted mind, "Well, might as well get high since you feel well now," and it just started progressing again.

Nick's story is representative of many addicts' experiences. In the midst of addiction, they are obsessed with the process of getting high to where they have no consideration for others. It's not necessarily a conscious choice, to say to oneself "I'm going to wake up today and continue to put my family through hell." It just sort of happens. When it does, apathy is largely the only response they are capable of.

This OD was different. Being pronounced dead and having his most direct confrontation with his mortality made him reconsider his path. Throughout his decades of use, his loved ones had tried to get him to quit countless times to no avail. He didn't want to hear it. He wasn't ready. Waking up under a white sheet, recognizing the anguish he was causing the people he loved proved to be the moment, at the time, that finally broke through. Nevertheless, he kept using. For Nick, this overdose was the eye of the storm, a fleeting moment of clarity that would soon see him return to the same mess he'd grown accustomed to. He did so almost reluctantly, but the more he used the more he remembered why he loved it in the first place. He couldn't resist the temptation of going from only getting well to getting high. Still, the empathy that he felt for his family in the aftermath of his last overdose, combined with his first true instance of critical self-reflection, marked the point where he began to recognize that if he kept using it was going to kill him for good. For the first time, he was scared. Eventually, it played a significant role in his decision to get clean.

One of Tim's (WM33) overdoses was also a wake-up call. Though, like Nick, it didn't immediately stop him from using. In the moment, it was just like any of his other three ODs. He almost died, but didn't, so he kept getting high. He wasn't yet moved by the significance of what transpired. In the months after, as his life increasingly began to fall apart, his reflection on the timing of that last OD weighed on him immensely,

> I woke up. They said that they had to give me Narcan four times. It was the first time I ever had Narcan. They gave it to me twice in the nose, and then twice in a shot in my veins. I woke up drenched in sweat. When I came to, I was very disoriented. I was very dehydrated. I couldn't walk. I was just fucked up. Not high, just very disoriented. You would have thought that it would have slowed my use down. It didn't. The last one, I didn't even think about it, but it was two days after my son's birthday. I look back, I OD'd two days after my son's birthday. He just turned four. I don't know. It just makes me wonder what the fuck I'm doing. I'm selfish to not think of him. He's so young. I never had a father. For me to fucking OD or to show him, to lead by that example…That should be a happy time, he just had a birthday. We should be celebrating his birthday. I don't know, so many different feelings and ideas and thoughts about that one resonated. I mean, it did. Why? I don't really know why that one out of the other ones did,

because I still had my son prior, but it did. I've thought about it a lot…But I continued to get high after that. It wasn't for too much longer, though.

When Tim tried to get clean, the proximity of his overdose to his son's birthday was one of, if not the greatest motivator he had for seeing it through. Dwelling on that few days-long period was the epitome a "spoiled self" (McIntosh and McKeageny 2002). He'd experienced not having a father and it was the last thing he wanted for his son, which meant he needed to "get his shit together because he couldn't be there for his son if he was dead." Tim admitted that not running from treatment was a daily struggle. He'd ran before. Four out of five times, to be exact. This time was different. Internally, he had a true desire to stay clean, something that he lacked in each prior instance.

Nothing Could Make Me Stop But Me

> *When you get in trouble or if your family is pressuring you, I've been to treatment so many times, I can tell you what you want to hear. I can make it sound so…We are master manipulators; we are master liars. We are great at it. I could probably make people believe anything I said. I'm really good at it, but honestly, especially when I'm doing it to appease somebody else, you can't trust what I'm saying. I truly believe the only person that will ever know when you're ready is you, and I even feel like sometimes the desire is there. If you would have asked me when I went to treatment, if I was going to use again, you could have hooked me up to a lie detector and I would have said no and I would have passed, and yet I got out and used two days later…They would be telling you the truth when they said, "I don't ever want to get high again. I want to stay clean." And then they're dead three days later.*

> *- Michelle (WF28)*

By and large, addicts cannot be forced, shamed, or court-ordered into staying clean– it simply doesn't work. They can be provided with all of the opportunities in the world (Giordano et al. 2002), but external pressures are not sufficient to negate the internal drive of a drug-addicted mind and body seeking to perpetuate the cycle of use. Family distress, mounting arrests, time spent incarcerated, or even knocking on death's door cannot dissuade an addict from using unless they have a desire to change. Despite what some might hypothesize regarding other forms of crime (Laub and Sampson 1993; Massoglia and Uggen 2010; Sampson and Laub 1990; Uggen 2000), the presence or absence of social bonds bore little influence over addicts' desire to use. Loved ones quickly recognized that their desperate pleas to stop or to get help didn't work. In response to their unwillingness to quit, addicts' loved ones or concerned parties had decisions to make regarding how they would approach the problem. Responses typically resembled two options– compassionate absentee support or by issuing ultimatums.

As her addiction worsened, Liz's (AF34) family adopted the former. Liz struggled with addiction since she was 17. We met her earlier, when we discussed her experiences making trips down to Florida to cover her habit after her enabling grandparents died. Her use was nearly constant, with two brief periods of sobriety somewhere in there– she couldn't recall exactly when. While she's never been through a formal rehab program, concerned family, despite strained relationships, tried on numerous occasions to get her clean and off the streets. None of those attempts influenced her desire to use, necessitating a modified approach,

> *Within yourself, you have to want it, and nobody can want it for you.* You have to want it…My mom and my dad, of course, my sister, my kids. I can't even do it for my kids. My children, they would see me prostitute myself on the street. It burned my heart. But my kids didn't understand the nature of the disease. My family would see me walking on the street, stop and pick me up, and go get me

something to eat, get me a pack of cigarettes, and then let me out. I just wasn't ready, and they knew that, and they say, "When you're ready, we're ready." Once I got that concept, everything started changing. People started changing, like my mom, my sister, my kids, my dad. People's hearts started softening and now I know that I'm a part of this family that now they want something to do with me.

Liz knew that nothing they did would change her mind. The presence of persistent hooks for change– regaining her family's support, her children, and the resources they had lined up for her– made no difference (Giordano et al. 2002). She had not yet reached a point where *she* wanted to stop using. There was nothing that was going to make her stop. She loathed herself for doing what she was. Never in a million years did she think she'd be selling herself. Worse, that her daughter would watch it happen. After numerous intrusive failed attempts, her family adopted a laissez-faire approach to her addiction. As difficult as it was, they came to recognize that the only path forward was to give her space and that when she was ready, they would support her recovery. Until then, they accepted the hard reality that they must wait for her addiction to run its course and hope she survived.

In other instances, loved ones took a more hardline approach, nearly always to disastrous, ineffective results. After decades of using a cornucopia of drugs, Keith's (WM45) family was well-accustomed to his modus operandi. He'd pop up whenever he needed money and they were lucky if any given run at sobriety to get someone off his back was even half-hearted. It didn't stop them from trying. To him, it didn't matter if the task of getting clean had been court-ordered either– if anyone pushed too hard, they ran the risk of having him pull away with even greater force,

It was either to keep the judge off my back, or because the court ordered. Maybe it made my mom happy, or my grandma happy. Keep my wife's mouth shut, or do it for my kids, but for myself? No. I had no desire to. I was doing what I wanted to do. I was getting high, that's all I cared about…Because in the end I got the ultimate say of what I do. You know what I mean? Whether it's to stay clean, or to keep using. You can hold whatever you want to hold…You hold your intervention all you want. I'll sit there and listen to all you guys bitching, and whine, and complain, but when you're done, I'm going to go out there and I'm going to stick a needle in my arm. I'm going to do it for one reason only: and that's to piss you off. I would've for spite because you held an intervention on me.

Heroin was different than crack and meth. Those were his drugs of choice up until the past few years when opioids took over. Somehow, he was even more obstinate now than he used to be. Keith wanted everyone to leave him alone and let him do his drugs in peace. They persisted, but only further alienated him in the process.

Issuing ultimatums was a near-certain route to temporary placation and eventual relapse. When his use of percs started to be a problem, Todd's (WM36) girlfriend told him to shape up or they were done. He was starting to get sloppy, nodding out at home in full view of her young children. His behavior was also becoming increasingly erratic, staying out all night and disappearing for days at a time. Todd knew she was right; he needed help, but he didn't want it, "My girlfriend gave me an ultimatum that if I didn't stop and go check into treatment that she was leaving. [I] Played along for a little bit. Probably five years. She tolerated my shit for a few years… I don't think that helped. I was sneaking around using two weeks later. I still felt like shit. I didn't want to have to keep using them [pills] like that. I didn't want to have to keep spending the money. A lot of fucking money." All treatment and her threats did was make his use more covert. Physical pain from a work injury coupled with withdrawal symptoms had him locked into using. The hard reality was that she didn't matter to him as much as opioids did. She was a clear-cut secondary priority.

In either instance, whether hands-off compassion or hardline orders, the result was likely a disappointment to users' loved ones. When an addict tried to get clean for them, it didn't work. They wanted to want the same things as their families, but they didn't, at least not yet. Motivations for trying were typically associated with the desire of easing the burden on concerned, estranged family, as in Linda's (WF33) case. Her earliest attempts at getting off heroin stemmed from her desire to please her family. She felt guilty for what her addiction put them through and what it did to her children. At her worst, she still maintained a sense of obligation she felt towards them, but opioids were pulling her in the opposite direction,

> I think the first few times I was doing it just for my family. I still wanted to get high, but my family didn't want me to get high no more and wanted me home with my kids and stuff. So, I was like, "All right, whatever. I'll go [to treatment]." So, I went, and something would happen, or I'd make something up, and I would leave. I would never complete it. Because I wasn't ready. But this time, because of all the stuff from before and everything that had ever happened to me being on the streets, I was done. I was totally done. And I was doing it for me this time…I'd say a good five years was how long it took.

As badly as her family wanted her to quit, for both her safety and their own peace of mind, they could only do so much. Several attempts orchestrated to deliver her at various rehab programs sputtered. Without a court order, they weren't compulsory; if she wanted to leave, the facility couldn't stop her. It was only after five years of living life on the streets that she had endured enough trauma to want to try to get clean. She finally recognized her feared self and knew she had to stop (Paternoster and Bushway 2009).

The desire to get clean for the sake of one's family was goal-oriented in other instances, motivated by a need to get something back that was being withheld from them. For example, an addicted mother's objective was often focused on regaining custody of her children. Still, the process of desisting was often untenable. In Anna's (WF28) case, her history of substance use and her recent introduction to the power of IV heroin use proved to be too powerful to overcome.

After suffering numerous instances of sexual abuse as a pre-teen, Anna turned to drugs and alcohol to work her way through the confusion. Her parents were also users and were never a sure thing to be present, let alone stop her from using substances. She struggled through life, trying to deal with the obstacles that her addictions created. After her husband passed, her infant son was the only true family she had in her life. When her heroin use worsened and she became homeless, her ability to be a fit parent was compromised, compelling child services to intervene. She was crushed to lose custody of him, but still could not bring herself to quit using. She tried, on numerous occasions, but her desire to get him back was no match for her need to chase dope,

> I wasn't ready. I was doing it for somebody else. I was doing it because I missed my son and I wanted that relationship with him, but that wasn't enough. I had to want it for me because heroin has a grip on you. *It's the only thing that's more powerful than my son and I had to be completely ready to let go.* It's like a relationship. You can't live with it, can't live without it. I was tired of the way I was living. I was tired of being sick and doing things that I was doing, but them first three days [of withdrawals]– I have to remember them first three days because they were...it was hell. That was hell. There's times still today where I'm like "I want it, I miss it. I miss the feeling. I miss the process. I miss the lifestyle. I miss it," but treatment thankfully has taught me coping skills where I have to take a breath and remember those three days because those three days are what brought me here...I have to remember the last month that I was out there. I remember the good times. I like to always remember the good times. You forget the bad. You glorify it. I always have to remember just in case.

Now sober, Anna is able to fully comprehend the magnitude of her addiction. Her inability to quit in order to regain her son caused her immense guilt, but it wasn't enough. She tried to stop, and she had been exposed to treatment and the same coping skills that are aiding her now, but neither, in and of themselves, was capable of helping her maintain sobriety. She had to hit her breaking point first. Ultimately, the trauma she endured has become a silver lining of sorts. The memories of her life on the street, of having to sell herself, and of the violence she experienced, serve as a counterweight to remaining urges to start the cycle again. Whenever she has a craving, she's able to recall what it felt like to live in hell. She focuses on remembering her bottom and how finding her internal breaking point marked the beginning of the end.

I Didn't Care if I Lived or Died

There's a reason why addicts refer to a bottom with as much resignation as they do. After chasing dope day-in day-out, many find it hard to muster the desire to want to keep going even though their bodies demand it. They're trapped in a cycle where self-loathing and physical distress are the norm. Often times, false bottoms feature many of the same events as the final one– thefts, sickness, etc., but true indifference to death was often an indicator of the recognition of a feared self and the final bottom (Paternoster and Bushway 2009). Most addicts reported experiencing at least one period where they recalled experiencing extreme depression or no longer having the will to live. For some, they were outright suicidal, but most had more of a "if it happens, it happens" mentality. The notion of dying didn't seem all that bad. It might even be a blessing, they thought. Existing in that frame of mind for prolonged periods did damage to their psyches, serving as a significant, consistent component of the process of bottoming out.

Steve (WM44), he of three overdoses and a broken ankle in a grocery store bathroom, wasn't suicidal, but dying wasn't a problem. He'd been living through what he thought were a series of worsening bottoms for too long to care anymore. Once the owner of several successful small businesses, he was completely destitute. Fast forward through several years spent living on the streets, and Steve was tapped out,

> Oh, yeah– I hit rock bottom. I slept on the streets before. I've been in abandonds [houses]. I've been in crazy shit. Stuff that I care not to even to talk about. It was bad. Real bad. Fight for your life at night, shoot outs. I mean, crazy…It got bad that I didn't care if I lived or died. It was hit bottom, get comfortable. That's most people's stories though… Was years, man. "Who cares?" "Today could be my day." "This might be my last day. I'll just go all out every day." I wasn't feeling nothing. You know what I mean?...I don't know if anyone could have helped me. I really don't know. I can't honestly tell you yes or no. I think at that point the only thing I was going to have to have was a spiritual awakening like I did. I think that's the only thing that would've saved my life, I really do. I don't think that anybody could have told me anything. I was that far gone…In order for recovery to work, you got to want it. With anything, you got to go after it, you got to go get it. The real turning point was ODing and being dead for 22 minutes. It just woke me up, man. It really did. I don't even know...I felt different, man, when I woke up. I care a lot more. I really do.

Twenty-two minutes. Steve was pronounced dead and woke up 22 minutes later. After one minute, brain cells begin to die. After five, death becomes imminent. After 15, survival is nearly impossible. Steve? He's just fine. Lucid, talkative, engaging; he's all there. He was beyond fortunate to emerge from the incident as he did. As a reminder of the ordeal, he has one of the documents from that night framed on his wall, not that he needs help remembering.

Before that moment, dying wouldn't have mattered to Steve. That was his daily mindset and he lived it for years; it became normal. He'd had several overdoses before this. There were plenty of friends and family that wished he would quit, and they made it known too. Time and time again, and counter to some conventional perspectives expectations (Sampson and Laub

1993), his connections to others couldn't change his mind. He was determined to keep using, regardless of anyone else's wants or desires. It took one momentous act to set him on a new course of his choosing. He felt as if he hit his true personal bottom. He now knew he was ready to stop. As some theorists would expect (Paternoster and Bushway 2009), it was his fear of what continuing living the same life would mean that was the key. This time, as opposed to those prior, dying made him want to live. From past failures, he understood the importance of caring about recovery and the need to be fully committed. There was a time when Steve couldn't go 22 minutes without thinking about getting high, but now, he never wants to go back to that life.

After over ten years of use, there was hardly a bridge left that Jessica (WF35) hadn't burned. She'd fallen into the trap of trying to quit for others several times. She was able to keep it up for a while, but those episodes inevitably ended with a relapse. The failures only made things worse for her. She would wonder why the people she tried to stay sober for weren't enough for it to happen, pushing her deeper into depression and heroin use. The simple answer was that she wasn't ready yet. It took reaching a point where Jessica felt like she couldn't fall any further to finally relent,

> I was so depressed that I was praying to God that every shot would be my last. It got that way. Life was just got so miserable, it felt like it would be better to not be– I had felt like I had lost my soul. I felt like a soulless being. I felt like everything I touched, I destroyed. I felt like the drugs weren't even working anymore. There was nothing that could make me feel like I mattered. I felt like I had done so much shit in my life that there was no way people could possibly forgive me for it. I felt like I would never amount to nothing. It was the saddest time of my life. I stole from my grandmother. I cheated on my kids' dad a lot. I lost my kids. My kids weren't even enough for me to stop using. I hung out with people that did really terrible things to people. I stole from everywhere I went, I

lied to everyone I knew, nothing I did was good. Everything I did was so that I could get more drugs. I was in autopilot and I just would do anything I had to do to get the drugs that I needed.

I feel like I finally surrendered. I didn't have any warrants or anything. I told the police, "Please, just take me to the hospital man. I'll just figure it out from there." [Now] I have a relationship with my 13-year-old daughter. We talk quite a bit…It means everything to me. I know that it's going to be hard and I know that it's not going to happen overnight. But I know that it's something that can happen as long as I'm working a consistently solid program.

Her suicidal thoughts were symptoms of the damage she created during her descent. Once part of a tightly-knit family, Jessica was completely alone. Having failed at maintaining those relationships and wondering how she would ever get clean with the guilt she carried, there was nothing in her life but hopelessness. However, after reaching a breaking point, Jessica was able to commit to rehabilitation and focus on the small steps necessary begin to work on herself. She knew it wasn't going to be easy, but her personal desire to do better gave her a sense of determination she hadn't had in years.

Just Tired… Just Completely Exhausted

A crucial component of the process of reaching a breaking point and changing thinking was the arrival at a point of complete and utter exhaustion. In many ways, the expression of these feelings heavily overlapped with the urge to die; however, that was not always the case. For some, exhaustion was the primary component to desistance, even if they had thought about death. Sooner or later, the lifestyle that the pursuit of opioids necessitates takes a toll on an addict. They reach the point where, often over the course of several years of addiction, there is no longer enjoyment in drug use. As tolerances escalate, the volume of drugs they require

186

increases. They find themselves not only chasing a fleeting high, but also the funds to do so, often contributing to elevated levels of criminal activity and increased exposure to physical harm.

After years spent in addiction, Christine (WF31) came to the realization that she couldn't continue. Too much had happened. She'd experienced enough trauma and loss to where anything more seemed unfathomable (Paternoster and Bushway 2009). The sum of everything that had transpired while she was in her addiction, the majority of which happened after she switched to heroin, had worn her down to nothing,

> I was just fed up, tired. I didn't even give a fuck. Actually, I feel like maybe part of me wanted to die. Just tired. I was tired. I was tired of people ripping me off. I was tired...I started getting dope sick then. I was so tired of the life. I was just ran down. I had some incidents, like where I've been raped on the streets. It just got bad. I was just really tired. I went through a lot. I had a guy pull a knife on me and leave me out in the country. I've been in fights, been ripped off. I went to jail a couple times. It was just everything. I was so tired. But it seemed like when I did the heroin, that's when everything got worse.

She was going to die. It was that simple. She lost everything fairly quickly, but it took living in that state and enduring trauma after trauma for everything to finally click. The emotional pain of the loss of personal relationships– custody of her children, and the death of her father– motivated her drug use as she sought to numb the pain. Throughout those binges, she was also numbing her ability to recognize the physical trauma she was experiencing.

Anna (WF28) was one of the women that initially tried to get clean in the attempt to regain custody of her child, only to fail. As she continued to use, she knew that if she got clean she would have them back, but the draw of those bonds weren't enough to make her consider quitting (Giordano et al. 2002; Sampson and Laub 1993). She still had an internal desire to use. It took her reaching a point where, like Christine, she had decided that she had suffered enough. Mentally and physically broken, she knew she had to be done. If she didn't stop, she was afraid that she would die. When I asked what it was that finally made her say "enough," she recalled the negative experiences that, in sum, broke through,

> Rape, being held hostage for 13 hours one time, two days another time. Just being sick and tired of being sick and tired. It got to the point where I couldn't even perform [prostituting]. I was too paranoid that I was going to die from trying to make money. It's like a control thing because addicts, we don't have no control, so we try to control things. If I was going to die, I wanted to go out the way I wanted to go out, not by a man's hands. I don't know. I was homeless. I wasn't making a lot of money because I lost a lot of things. I was struggling to maintain my habit and finding a place to sleep, hotels with a John. Or on the streets. It was bad…I was overdosing left and right that last week.

Anna recognized that she was no longer in control. Previously, when she would make half-hearted attempts to get clean, there was a sense that she "could just stop." However misguided, she still felt as if she had agency. What she had yet to realize was that that mindset, minimizing the strength of the opponent she was facing, was sabotaging her efforts to get clean. Even throughout the tricking, stealing, and beatings, contrary to reality, she retained the notion that she could walk away when she needed to. If she was honest with herself, that moment had long since passed. It was only after she recognized and acknowledged her extreme fatigue and the deterioration of her situation that she fully committed to seeking help.

Others reached a similar point of exhaustion, but one that was primarily rooted in emotional fatigue. Mike (WM34) was a functional addict for several years. He worked as a chef when he started selling percs on the side for some extra cash. Curiosity got the best of him, they got expensive, and he went to heroin. He didn't want to, but he couldn't work when he was sick,

> There's this quote, it's like, "When your pain outweighs your desire to change." That's what it was for me. The whole entire time, I didn't wanna be a drug addict. Even a lot of it, I enjoyed the drugs for the first half, but then the second half, I didn't. I was just like...Just being dope-sick...I just didn't wanna be dope-sick and I wanted to keep my jobs and do everything. It stopped becoming fun. There's no longer like, "I wanna do drugs to get high." It was like, "I need to do drugs, so I'm not dope-sick." But all that pain, it finally just got to the point where it's just like…I'm stopping because I'm tired of this hurt and I'm tired of the pain. Even though I always wanted to change, I didn't really want to change. I wanted to change, but I wanted it to come easy. And I think I finally just got to the point where it's just like, "This isn't gonna be easy to overcome, but I'm just tired of it."

By the time he graduated to heroin, drugs were no longer fun. Addiction was a burden. When he still enjoyed them, he tried stopping. A couple times for his family, a couple times for a girl. None of the attempts lasted long. He even tried suboxone, but that led straight back to heroin– it was considerably cheaper. Through the lens of "I want to quit," Mike justified using so he could stay functional and keep working. He could only do that for so long before things truly fell apart and he found himself living in his car. Once consequences began to mount, he grew weary of the routine and arrived at what he regards as his bottom. From that point, he embraced a long-term treatment program, eventually obtaining gainful employment and several years of sobriety.

Not everyone's breaking point was the same. Relative to others, Angela (WF33) had it good. There's no minimizing what she went through on a personal level, but she was fortunate that she had the foresight to recognize the warning signs earlier than most. Her burnout and fatigue weren't masked by opioids like many others'. Instead, they alerted her to what was in store for her if she persisted, motivating a change,

> I'm just drained from all of it. Because I took a look at my aunt and she's like 55 years old, still doing drugs, looks like she's on drugs. It's just bad. All you see is bones and no teeth, and super tiny. And I'm like, "I just don't want to be like that." Her kids don't really like her anymore because they reflect on how things were growing up. I'm just like, "That's not who I want to be." And we look too much alike. If she had meat on her bones, I would look like her. And I'm like, "I know if I continue, that's what I'm going to look like. And I can't do that." But I just reflected on that. Like, I can't…that's one of the first things I always thought about.

Angela had a glimpse into the future. Her feared self sat immediately before her. She saw what that life would entail if she persisted, and it was enough to make her want to embrace change. She couldn't look like that, couldn't permanently alienate her kids, and couldn't be that broke forever. It was an alternate reality that she had to avoid at all costs.

"Too Old For This Shit": Long-term Use and The Emergence of Latent Maturity

For long-term addicts, a key component of addiction-related fatigue was intimately tied to the recognition of the longevity of their use. In a sense, they were a small sub-set of individuals that had "aged out" of using (Hirschi and Gottfredson 1983; Massoglia and Uggen 2010). Importantly, there was no common age threshold in this respect. Rather, the subjective notion of "advanced age" was a fluid concept tied largely to duration of use– someone in their late-20s could express the same sentiments as someone in their late-40s. Irrespective of age, the longer an addict lives the life that typically accompanies chasing opioids, the older they feel. On the heels of years of addiction, many had a moment of clarity where they realized they had been

190

using for too long. I mentioned John (WM36) when I talked about differences in every addict's bottom. A user of roughly 13 years, he was never fazed by seeing another addict sleeping in a cardboard box. Getting clean was a long time coming. For others, he said, hitting bottom could be as simple as seeing someone else at a low point, similar to how Angela viewed her aunt. Alternatively, it might get ugly. John knew the difference; he fell into the latter category. When he bottomed out, and stayed there, it eventually took recognizing that he was no longer as resilient to the difficulties of street life as he once had been,

> What it was is just as I got older, I could see myself, where it was taking me again. I would just slowly regulate it, or slowly try to quit, which, in the past, I never did that. I would just go on runs; I would take it all the way until it put me in jail or whatever. I didn't care what I did, but as I've just gotten older, it's just gotten old. You just get tired of jail and living on the streets and shit like that, so I would just try to control it myself, or wean myself down, and off. That's why I would just go to rehab so much, or even when I would go to rehab, I would just lay in bed until it passed, and I could start eating Suboxone. I just got sick and tired of being sick and tired. Took me like 13 years… I'm tired of sitting in the fucking hood, and I'm tired of being broke. Most of it is that I'm tired of my life literally revolving around one thing. I wake up, I have to have this. I got to go get more money to have this, I got to make sure I have enough when I wake up to have this. It's literally, that's all your brain thinks about is having one thing. And there's more to life than just that. It just gets old, of just the same thing, day-in and day-out, you know? It's miserable.

The misery of the daily grind of chasing dope every day for over a decade was immeasurable. By the end, John had been through the cycle of trying to stop and failing enough to know when he was truly spent. In each of the times prior to this one, detoxing was the brief respite he needed to recover. Once he had, it was back out to the streets to do it all over again. The drive to pursue dope still hadn't relented, but after so many years, he finally broke.

Ryan (WM49) came to a similar realization. Thirteen years John's senior, Ryan started young, his first period of addiction taking place in the early 1980s, placing him among the longest-tenured users in my sample. With roughly six periods of use and two stints in rehab, he'd been clean off and on. Granted, his heart wasn't fully in it either time he tried to stop. A rough childhood, evidenced by his pre-teen drug addiction, left lasting marks that marred his development. Drugs were always the outlet. Normatively, using was almost expected in his environment and "staying fucked up" became his default. It took decades to break that cycle for good, or at least for the longest time he's had since he started,

> My age. I just, I've done it for so long. Once I really cleared my head of just how unhappy I was, just didn't like what I was. I'm just now starting to learn to like and love myself. I just, something I've never really dealt with from earlier issues. Just tired, just got sick and tired of it. And since I've been working on my spiritual part of my program, my higher power…I just feel, all my experiences are some type of purpose. There's a greater purpose of what God wants me to do, and just letting him lead me to where that's going to be here. Just how the streets are so deadly now, I don't think I have another chance to go back out there and start using and make it back alive. I'm seeing the benefits of cleaning myself up, feeling better about myself, getting happy. I mean truly happy for, I can't remember when I was really, really, truly happy, it's been so long. Feeling good about myself. Just confidence…Knowing there's some type of purpose, and as I'm doing the right thing, things are falling into place for me. So, I'm getting the rewards of sobriety. And I see it in other people in the rooms, AA and NA, people who have longer sobriety, they all say that they've been blessed with the things they need.

Getting clean wasn't a pit stop this time. As Paternoster and Bushway (2009) would expect, it was a moment of clarity that permitted the recognition of the toll his use had taken on him after using for so long. His view of what the future held finally scared him enough to accept that change was necessary. It had become unavoidable.

Part of the salience of age was not just the relation it often had to exhaustion. Many related their changes in thinking to developing maturity or the aspiration to be more mature. They could no longer afford to engage in what they regarded as juvenile behavior if they were going to turn their lives around. Donte (BM40) was an active drug seller as far back as he could remember. He and his associates would dabble in whatever they were selling, but percs became something more than that. He quickly developed a physical dependency and switched over to heroin once the pills became scarce. Donte had several children at this point. He had always been an active parent. He believed in the importance of being present in their lives and valued the role he played in shaping them as they grew, a responsibility that was sidetracked by opioids,

> When you become older, you start to put away foolish childish things, do grownup stuff. You ain't got too much because 18, 19 years old, hell you've got more years to find your way. You got plenty of chances. Now, you just need to tighten up. That's how I look at it, just like children getting older. You've got to set a better example. When they wasn't here, you wouldn't worry about nothing like that, so that's what it is for me…That's your offspring. You want to leave a positive legacy, you know? At least you don't want your kids to start repeating what you do, so you just want to change it up. Them getting older, what they think of you, that's who you are to them.

Internally, Donte had a sense for what was acceptable adult behavior and what wasn't. When he was younger, he was just messing around, being a young adult trying different things. Once opioids began, the things that were important to him became background noise. When he was focused on heroin, there was no room to focus on anything else. By the time he hit 40, he knew his time was up. Emblematic of Massoglia and Uggen's (2010) study of the barriers that crime present to progress into adulthood, Donte knew that living the life of an addict stood in the way of being anything more. His kids were getting older and were entering the stages of life where they could start making the same mistakes that he had at that age, an outcome he desperately wanted to avoid. He knew that in order to play the role of a well-intentioned parent effectively and have any credibility with his kids, he had to grow up and get clean.

Ron (WM37) started using in his early 20s and has had trouble stringing together legitimate periods of sobriety ever since. Twice he was able to get a few weeks before he turned 25, but that was all. Between 25 and the present, it was nothing but using. Over the course of those years, he was no stranger to trouble. He'd been arrested somewhere around ten times, all for drugs. Percs, heroin, fetty– you name it, he'd done it,

> I'm 37 years old. it's time to grow the hell up. I've thrown away a lot of good opportunities. I've been strung out for a long time and I'm just like, "I'm tired of being tired." I know that I can have a lot more in life, I want more in life than to be strung out sleeping on the floor or someone's couch. So, I came here at first and I had a "fuck it" attitude about this. I was gonna say, "I'll fucking leave"…but one day, things just started clicking. I've had a whole different attitude, like happy to be here…try and put all this behind me.

Now, Ron has a job and works 60 hours a week. Back then, he exhibited what Giordano et al. (2002) would expect to be the necessary perspective to succeed in recovery– he was willing to try. On several occasions, he tried to capitalize on the opportunities that were afforded to him, but the allure of working a straight job or maintaining connections to family were incompatible with his continued desire to use. It was only after he decided that he was through using that those opportunities, ones that he's beginning to take advantage of now, had a chance to help change his life. He's excelling for the first time in as long as he can remember and the satisfaction he derives from knowing how far he's come since that fateful moment where he said "I'm too old for this" helps keep him on track.

A consistent component of the aging narrative was the feeling of having lost time to addiction. By expending so much energy on an all-consuming, unproductive task, addicts would often reflect on how little had truly happened over the course of their addictions. For example, Kelly (WF27), thinking about her 11 years of opioid use, recognized that her life had stagnated,

> I feel like I've literally done nothing in 10 years but be an addict. I've had times of being clean but it's like, I don't even remember those. I only remember the bad parts of when I'm using. And I literally feel like I'm in the same spot. I don't even feel like I'm 27. I feel like I'm 16 still. I feel like I'm the same age because my life hasn't progressed in any way. I'm at the same spot as I was back then and I'm getting too old to be doing this shit. I should be way further along in life and I'm almost 30 years old.

Developing a full-fledged addiction at 16 put Kelly up against the odds that she was going to have a normal life as she got older, but she didn't realize how significant of an impact her addiction would have. It was almost as if the last ten years never happened. Heroin had stunted her personal development completely, such that she had nothing to show for the years that had passed in the interim. Although only 27, Kelly recognized that the clock was ticking; she had to break the pattern now before it was too late. The thought of arriving at 30 feeling 16 necessitated a change, so much so that it fostered a new sense of determination to avoid that outcome at all costs.

Conclusion: Striking a Balance

Amidst the continued impact of the opioid epidemic, this book has sought to investigate addicts' initiation, escalation, and cessation of opioid use in order to better inform.policy perspectives and assess the applicability and utility of criminological theory. First, to provide context, I detailed how many individuals' addictions can be traced back to unchecked access to prescription opioid painkillers, often involving elaborate interstate doctor shopping operations and pill mill exploitation. Whether obtained through legal or illicit means, fundamental flaws surrounding the dispersal of pills allowed individuals to quickly develop addictions. Changing regulations and the closure of medical loopholes generated widespread desperation among addicts as pills became increasingly scarce. Borne out of necessity, many addicts transitioned to heroin use to combat withdrawal symptoms.

This switch was often accompanied by escalations in criminal involvement. In the context of a justice system that frequently favors rigorous sanctions, I explored the suitability of deterrence-based principles for the policing of opioid addicts (Becker 1968; Kessler and Levitt 1999; Wilson and Boland 1978). As users' chemical dependencies worsened, addicts were increasingly incapable of performing the internal calculus that rational choice theory is predicated upon. Absent the capacity to properly weigh risk versus reward, addicts formed a deep indifference to the threat of criminal justice contact. Further, justice contact, in the form of arrest and/or incarceration, did little to dissuade users from pursuing their addictions, nor did it influence their desistance from crime.

Based on this finding, I examine the most salient factors contributing to addicts' respective decisions to get clean and the extent to which their thinking aligned with criminological theories on cognitive change (Giordano et al. 2002; Paternoster and Bushway

2009). Posing challenges for policy development, addicts described the inability of social bonds, such as marriage, family ties, or employment, to impact their motivation to continue opioid use (Sampson and Laub 1993). Instead, my findings indicate that lasting pursuits of sobriety were preceded by the organic development of an internal conviction to get clean. This decision was often closely tied to several factors, including the recognition of a personal "bottom," extreme physical and mental exhaustion, and a fear of the consequences of continued opioid use.

The severity and character of everyone's ultimate bottom was different, but every addict reached a turning point in their addiction where they said "enough." Counter to the expectations of deterrence theory, any interaction with police and the courts was merely a speed bump on the road to feeding ongoing opioid addictions, undermining the plausibility of specific deterrence in this case (Anwar and Loughran 2011; Matsueda et al. 2006; Pogarsky and Piquero 2003). Justice contact was only meaningful in the sense that it was but one component of a greater patchwork of undesirable circumstances. Even then, as shown, punitive punishment remained on the fringes of addicts' consciousness. An addict could be arrested 20 times and it would not matter. They could spend five years incarcerated, and similarly, it would not matter. In extreme cases, an addict could know with absolute certainty they would be apprehended for a crime, yet the drive to stay well negated any potential deterrent effect.

At best, a period of incarceration-induced sobriety provided an opportunity for the mental fog of opioid addiction to clear. After enduring withdrawals, many addicts described the process of making plans for after their release. They were often determined to "do better," and make the most of another chance at freedom. Ultimately, the promises that they made themselves while locked up rang hollow. The appeal of using again had an amnesia-like quality, erasing the memory of the consequences of their opioid use that had just concluded, sometimes only hours prior. With serious doubts concerning the efficacy of deterrence-inspired policing strategies, efforts must focus on the identification of alternatives.

Giordano et al. (2002) would likely expect that the pursuit of sobriety would begin with an openness to change. From that position, opportunities to pursue pro-social hooks for change would coax a user out of addiction as they increasingly formed conventional bonds. Indeed, many addicts expressed a desire to change. At times, uncertainty regarding the availability of resources made continuing addiction easier, despite the development of any misgivings with their lifestyle. Though, from a critical perspective, it is fair to wonder the degree to which this perspective applies to the cessation of opioid use. Most often, when an addict was open to alternative pathways, the presence of socially beneficial opportunities could not consistently influence change. Evidenced by the numerous instances of addicts bypassing treatment, eschewing court ordered aid, and the rejection of pleas from loved ones, a reliance on simply presenting alternatives, predicated on the assumption of an openness to them, is a naïve strategy.

More in line with Paternoster and Bushway (2009), I would argue that the frustrating, less-desirable route is most realistic. It is essential that the desistance process begins with an internal desire to change and an addict's recognition of a feared self. There must be a moment where the projected consequences of continuing ongoing addiction outweigh the desire to continue using, irrespective of the availability of pathways towards another life. Attempts to coerce addicts into cessation, even when well-intentioned, were often met with the reaction opposite of what was intended. Instead, addicts were often driven deeper into a defiant mindset where incurring additional harms out of spite was almost welcomed. If the sincere desire to get clean does not originate from within, and if opportunities or hooks for change do not come after that point, the prospect of achieving enduring sobriety is dubious at best.

198

I have shown that the underlying motivations for the decision to desist from opioid use are typically related to some form of burnout, but this knowledge does not provide much utility in a practical sense. The imperative to reduce crime and ensure public safety prohibits an overly passive approach to the policing of addiction that would cease efforts to arrest and incarcerate addicts. Simply, that will never happen, nor should it. Nevertheless, the opioid epidemic is not solely a criminal justice problem, but also a matter of public health.

I would assert that the answer lies somewhere in between these competing paradigms. Punishment motivated by the desire to force addicts into sobriety or to reinforce lessons of socially desirable behavior are ineffective. Alternatively, punishment with targeted objectives that more closely align with public health emphases may hold potential. If addicts are held for a minimum period of time that extends beyond the totality of withdrawals, the justice system will provide opportunities for addicts to critically reflect on their current state. At the same time, the offer of voluntary treatment resources would give providers the opportunity to interact with addicts and expose them to alternative paths, hopefully aiding in the cultivation of the desire to pursue change. However, it is important to temper expectations.

Along these lines, the pro-social hooks for change that Giordano et al.'s (2002) model would hope to leverage, while likely ineffective in the context of timid openness to change, can have utility in the proper circumstances. If presented in a passive fashion, addicts may internalize the existence of what an alternate path could resemble. In other words, it may be possible to "plant the seed" in addicts' minds that help exists, and it is available to them when they are ready. When the time comes that their disenchantment with addiction is nearing the tipping point of no longer being the preferred path forward, knowledge of pro-social opportunities may aid in making the decision to quit. Knowing concretely what the "first step" in recovery will be, as opposed to a nebulous conception of something "else," may be capable of reducing reservations and uncertainty, making the decision easier. In the absence of any kind of awareness of desirable alternatives, I would argue that the proverbial tipping point becomes harder to reach. Further, there is no harm in passively presenting alternatives, even if they precede an addict's internal conviction to get clean, albeit with the understanding that failure is overwhelmingly likely. In rare cases, an addict's response to avenues to a different life may more closely align with Giordano et al.'s (2002) expectations for desistance, acting as the impetus for change.

As my findings indicate, addicts must develop a resolute desire to change before any such resources are likely to support meaningful change. Coupled with the realities surrounding the high probability of relapse, the most efficacious strategy going forward will be prevention. In that sense, and as was the case amidst my sample, ignorance regarding the dangers associated with even short-term opioid use must be more widely known. Public awareness campaigns, in addition to thorough patient education efforts on the part of prescribers, may aid in reducing the number of individuals that follow to pill-to-heroin pathway.

Importantly, the make-up of my sample poses limitations. The racial composition of my sample is heavily White. It is important for future research to strive for increasingly diverse samples in order to assess and uncover differences in addiction experiences. Another potential limitation relates to eligibility criteria. In order to participate, an individual must have had some form of prior contact with the justice system. Although the vast majority of participants were involved in illegal activities beyond drug use prior to their first arrest, there may be noteworthy differences between individuals in my sample and others that have no arrest history. Lastly, as with most qualitative research, there are questions regarding the generalizability of my results, given the focus on one geographic location.

There are promising opportunities for future research to build off of this study. First, my data collection efforts are only a cross section in time. No additional data was collected after my interview with participants. Consequently, a lack of longitudinal data prohibits examinations of change over time. While my interviews probed participants' prior cycles of addiction, it would have been valuable to have the capacity to assess changes in attitudes and substance use over a period of observation. For example, in Adam's case, I was made aware of his passing as a result of circumstance. Without this knowledge, I would have assumed that he was likely living a life of sobriety, having so fully dedicated himself to his recovery. Sadly, that was not what transpired. Taken at his word, his opioid addiction was a thing of the past; a period of darkness that he had surmounted. He came to the realization that he could not continue on the same path and needed to change. He represents a sobering reminder of the inherent challenges of opioid recovery. An addict can do everything they were supposed to, but it still might not be enough.

The notion that the discovery of a breaking point or ultimate bottom will lead to lasting sobriety must be tempered. Instead, a breaking point should be thought of as a necessary, rather than sufficient condition. A wholehearted commitment to getting clean is still likely to result in relapse. Such is the nature of opioid addiction. Scenarios that see addicts achieve lasting sobriety are wishful thinking. One out of ten will make it one year without using after getting clean (Smyth et al. 2010). Beyond that year, there are no guarantees. Among my sample, on average, it took nearly seven attempts at getting clean before it stuck. In this case, that was typically for a period of roughly six months at the time of data collection, leaving half of a year for them to regress to the mean. While I will never know for certain, the odds are that many could not stay clean. For some, a relapse will be a momentary setback that becomes a footnote on a path to desistance. For others, it will mark the descent to yet another opioid-induced bottom and perhaps even their demise. Even still, we must continue to try.

References

Ahmed, Serge H. 2010. "Validation Crisis in Animal Models of Drug Addiction: Beyond Non-Disordered Drug Use toward Drug Addiction." *Neuroscience & Biobehavioral Reviews* 35(2):172–84.

Ahmed, Serge H., Magalie Lenoir, and Karine Guillem. 2013. "Neurobiology of Addiction versus Drug Use Driven by Lack of Choice." *Current Opinion in Neurobiology* 23(4):581–87.

Ahn, Woo-Young, Georgi Vasilev, Sung-Ha Lee, Jerome R. Busemeyer, John K. Kruschke, Antoine Bechara, and Jasmin Vassileva. 2014. "Decision-Making in Stimulant and Opiate Addicts in Protracted Abstinence: Evidence from Computational Modeling with Pure Users." *Frontiers in Psychology* 5.

Alexander, Michelle. 2012. *The New Jim Crow: Mass Incarceration in the Age of Colorblindness*. The New Press.

American Friends Service Committee. 1971. *Struggle for Justice: A Report on Crime and Punishment in America, Prepared for the American Friends Service Committee*. Hill & Wang.

Andenaes, Johannes. 1968. "Does Punishment Deter Crime Articles and Addresses." *Criminal Law Quarterly* 11(1):76–93.

Andenaes, Johannes. 1974. *Punishment and Deterrence*. University of Michigan Press.

Anglin, M. Douglas, and George Speckart. 1988. "Narcotics Use and Crime: A Multisample, Multimethod Analysis*." *Criminology* 26(2):197–233.

Anwar, Shamena, and Thomas A. Loughran. 2011. "Testing a Bayesian Learning Theory of Deterrence Among Serious Juvenile Offenders*." *Criminology* 49(3):667–98.

Apel, Robert. 2013. "Sanctions, Perceptions, and Crime: Implications for Criminal Deterrence." *Journal of Quantitative Criminology* 29(1):67–101.

Austin, James, John Clark, and Patricia Hardyman. 1998. *Three-Strikes and You're Out: The Implementation and Impact of Strike Laws*. Washington, D.C.: National Institute of Justice; U.S. Department of Justice.

Bachman, Ronet, Erin Kerrison, Raymond Paternoster, Daniel O'Connell, and Lionel Smith. 2016. "Desistance for a Long-Term Drug-Involved Sample of Adult Offenders: The Importance of Identity Transformation." *Criminal Justice and Behavior* 43(2):164–86.

Ball, John C., and Alan Ross. 2012. *The Effectiveness of Methadone Maintenance Treatment: Patients, Programs, Services, and Outcome*. Springer Science & Business Media.

Beccaria, Cesare. 1764. *On Crimes and Punishments*. 5th ed. Transaction Publishers.

Becker, Gary S. 1968. "Crime and Punishment: An Economic Approach." *Journal of Political Economy* 76(2):169–217.

Becker, Gary S., and Kevin M. Murphy. 1988. "A Theory of Rational Addiction." *Journal of Political Economy* 96(4):675–700.

Becker, Howard S. 1963. *Outsiders: Studies in the Sociology of Deviance*. Simon and Schuster.

Bennett, Trevor, and Katie Holloway. 2005. *Understanding Drugs, Alcohol And Crime*. McGraw-Hill Education (UK).

Bennett, Trevor, Katy Holloway, and David Farrington. 2008. "The Statistical Association between Drug Misuse and Crime: A Meta-Analysis." *Aggression and Violent Behavior* 13(2):107–18.

Bentham, Jeremy. 1789. *An Introduction to the Principles of Morals and Legislation*. HardPress.

Berger, Dan. 2014. *Captive Nation: Black Prison Organizing in the Civil Rights Era*. UNC Press Books.

Biernacki, Kathryn, Gill Terrett, Skye N. McLennan, Izelle Labuschagne, Phoebe Morton, and Peter G. Rendell. 2018. "Decision-Making, Somatic Markers and Emotion Processing in Opiate Users." *Psychopharmacology* 235(1):223–32.

Biernacki, Patrick. 1986. *Pathways from Heroin Addiction: Recovery Without Treatment.* Temple University Press.

Block, M. K., and J. M. Heineke. 1975. "A Labor Theoretic Analysis of the Criminal Choice." *The American Economic Review* 65(3):314–25.

Bluthenthal, Ricky N., Alex H. Kral, Elizabeth A. Erringer, and Brian R. Edlin. 1999. "A - Drug Paraphernalia Laws and Injection-Related Infectious Disease Risk among Drug Injectors." *Journal of Drug Issues* 29(1):1–16.

Bluthenthal, Ricky N., Alex Kral, Jennifer Lorvick, and John K. Watters. 1997. "Impact of Law Enforcement on Syringe Exchange Programs: A Look at Oakland and San Francisco." *Medical Anthropology* 18:61–83.

Bluthenthal, RickyN., Jennifer Lorvick, AlexH. Kral, ElizabethA. Erringer, and JamesG. Kahn. 1999. "B - Collateral Damage in the War on Drugs: HIV Risk Behaviors among Injection Drug Users." *International Journal of Drug Policy* 10(1):25–38.

Boles, Sharon M., and Karen Miotto. 2003. "Substance Abuse and Violence: A Review of the Literature." *Aggression and Violent Behavior* 8(2):155–74.

Bowling, Benjamin. 1999. "The Rise and Fall of New York Murder: Zero Tolerance or Crack's Decline?" *The British Journal of Criminology* 39(4):531–54.

Brady, Joanne E., Hannah Wunsch, Charles DiMaggio, Barbara H. Lang, James Giglio, and Guohua Li. 2014. "Prescription Drug Monitoring and Dispensing of Prescription Opioids." *Public Health Reports (1974-)* 129(2):139–47.

Braithwaite, John. 1989. *Crime, Shame and Reintegration.* Cambridge University Press.

Case, Anne, and Angus Deaton. 2015. "Rising Morbidity and Mortality in Midlife among White Non-Hispanic Americans in the 21st Century." *Proceedings of the National Academy of Sciences* 112(49):15078–83.

Chang, Hsien-Yen, Tatyana Lyapustina, Lainie Rutkow, Matthew Daubresse, Matt Richey, Mark Faul, Elizabeth A. Stuart, and G. Caleb Alexander. 2016. "Impact of Prescription Drug

Monitoring Programs and Pill Mill Laws on High-Risk Opioid Prescribers: A Comparative Interrupted Time Series Analysis." *Drug and Alcohol Dependence* 165:1–8.

Cheng, Erika R. 2012. "Disparities in Premature Mortality Between High- and Low-Income US Counties." *Preventing Chronic Disease* 9.

Chiricos, Ted, Kelle Barrick, William Bales, and Stephanie Bontrager. 2007. "The Labeling of Convicted Felons and Its Consequences for Recidivism*." *Criminology* 45(3):547–81.

Cicero, Theodore J., and Matthew S. Ellis. 2017. "The Prescription Opioid Epidemic: A Review of Qualitative Studies on the Progression from Initial Use to Abuse." *Dialogues in Clinical Neuroscience* 19(3):259–69.

Cooper, Hannah, Lisa Moore, Sofia Gruskin, and Nancy Krieger. 2005. "The Impact of a Police Drug Crackdown on Drug Injectors' Ability to Practice Harm Reduction: A Qualitative Study." *Social Science & Medicine* 61(3):673–84.

Corbin, Juliet, and Anselm Strauss. 2014. *Basics of Qualitative Research: Techniques and Procedures for Developing Grounded Theory.* SAGE Publications.

Corman, Hope, and H. Naci Mocan. 2000. "A Time-Series Analysis of Crime, Deterrence, and Drug Abuse in New York City." *The American Economic Review* 90(3):584–604.

Cushman, Paul Jr. 1974. "Relationship between Narcotic Addiction and Crime." *Federal Probation* 38:38.

"Council of Economic Advisers Report: The Underestimated Cost of the Opioid Crisis." *The White House.* Retrieved March 27, 2019 (https://www.whitehouse.gov/briefings-statements/cea-report-underestimated-cost-opioid-crisis/).

Daniels, Danni, Scott Grytdal, and Annemarie Wasley. 2009. "Surveillance for Acute Viral Hepatitis — United States, 2007." *Morbidity and Mortality Weekly Report: Surveillance Summaries* 58(3):1–27.

Daniulaityte, Raminta, Russel Falck, and Robert G. Carlson. 2012. "'I'm Not Afraid of Those Ones Just 'Cause They've Been Prescribed': Perceptions of Risk among Illicit Users of Pharmaceutical Opioids." *International Journal of Drug Policy* 23(5):374–84.

Dasgupta, Nabarun, Leo Beletsky, and Daniel Ciccarone. 2018. "Opioid Crisis: No Easy Fix to Its Social and Economic Determinants." *American Journal of Public Health* 108(2):182–86.

De Haan, Willem, and Jaco Vos. 2003. "A Crying Shame: The Over-Rationalized Conception of Man in the Rational Choice Perspective." *Theoretical Criminology* 7(1):29–54.

De Leon, George. 2000. *The Therapeutic Community: Theory, Model, and Method*. Springer Publishing Company.

De Maeyer, Jessica, Wouter Vanderplasschen, and Eric Broekaert. 2009. "Exploratory Study on Drug Users' Perspectives on Quality of Life: More than Health-Related Quality of Life?" *Social Indicators Research* 90(1):107–126.

De Maeyer, Jessica, Wouter Vanderplasschen, Jan Lammertyn, Chijs van Nieuwenhuizen, Bernard Sabbe, and Eric Broekaert. 2011. "Current Quality of Life and Its Determinants among Opiate-Dependent Individuals Five Years after Starting Methadone Treatment." *Quality of Life Research* 20(1):139–50.

Des Jarlais, Don C., Kamyar Arasteh, Salaam Semaan, and Evan Wood. 2009. "HIV among Injecting Drug Users: Current Epidemiology, Biologic Markers, Respondent-Driven Sampling, and Supervised-Injection Facilities." *Current Opinion in HIV and AIDS* 4(4):308–13.

Di Chiara, Gaetano. 2002. "Nucleus Accumbens Shell and Core Dopamine: Differential Role in Behavior and Addiction." *Behavioural Brain Research* 137(1):75–114.

Dietz, Thomas, and Tom R. Burns. 1992. "Human Agency and the Evolutionary Dynamics of Culture." *Acta Sociologica* 35(3):187–200.

Dom, Geert, Bieke De Wilde, Wouter Hulstijn, Wim Van Den Brink, and Bernard Sabbe. 2006. "Decision-Making Deficits in Alcohol-Dependent Patients With and Without Comorbid Personality Disorder." *Alcoholism: Clinical and Experimental Research* 30(10):1670–77.

Donroe, Joseph H., M. Eugenia Socias, and Brandon D. L. Marshall. 2018. "The Deepening Opioid Crisis in North America: Historical Context and Current Solutions." *Current Addiction Reports* 5(4):454–63.

Ehrlich, Isaac. 1972. "The Deterrent Effect of Criminal Law Enforcement." *The Journal of Legal Studies* 1(2):259–76.

Ehrlich, Isaac. 1973. "Participation in Illegitimate Activities: A Theoretical and Empirical Investigation." *Journal of Political Economy* 81(3):521–65.

Ehrlich, Isaac. 1975. "The Deterrent Effect of Capital Punishment: A Question of Life and Death." *The American Economic Review* 65(3):397–417.

Ekhtiari, Hamed, Teresa A. Victor, and Martin P. Paulus. 2017. "Aberrant Decision-Making and Drug Addiction—How Strong Is the Evidence?" *Current Opinion in Behavioral Sciences* 13:25–33.

Esterberg, Kristin G. 2002. *Qualitative Methods in Social Research*. McGraw-Hill.

Evans, William N., and Emily G. Owens. 2007. "COPS and Crime." *Journal of Public Economics* 91(1):181–201.

Farabee, David, Vandana Joshi, and M. Douglas Anglin. 2001. "Addiction Careers and Criminal Specialization." *Crime & Delinquency* 47(2):196–220.

Fareed, Ayman, Jungjin Kim, Bethany Ketchen, Woo Jin Kwak, Danzhao Wang, Hilaire Shongo-Hiango, and Karen Drexler. 2017. "Effect of Heroin Use on Changes of Brain Functions as Measured by Functional Magnetic Resonance Imaging, a Systematic Review." *Journal of Addictive Diseases* 36(2):105–16.

Fattah, Ezzat A. 1983. "A Critique of Deterrence Research with Particular Reference to the Economic Approach." *Canadian Journal of Criminology* 25(1):79–90.

Federation of State Medical Boards of the United States, Inc. 1998. *Model Guidelines for the Use of Controlled Substances for the Treatment of Pain.*

Fernández-Serrano, Maria Jose, Miguel Pérez-García, and Antonio Verdejo-García. 2011. "What Are the Specific vs. Generalized Effects of Drugs of Abuse on Neuropsychological Performance?" *Neuroscience & Biobehavioral Reviews* 35(3):377–406.

French, Michael T., Kerry Anne McGeary, Dale D. Chitwood, and Clyde B. McCoy. 2000. "Chronic Illicit Drug Use, Health Services Utilization and the Cost of Medical Care." *Social Science & Medicine* 50(12):1703–13.

Friedman, Samuel R., Enrique R. Pouget, Sudip Chatterjee, Charles M. Cleland, Barbara Tempalski, Joanne E. Brady, and Hannah L. F. Cooper. 2011. "Drug Arrests and Injection Drug Deterrence." *American Journal of Public Health* 101(2):344–49.

Gandossy, Robert P. 1980. *Drugs and Crime: A Survey and Analysis of the Literature.* Washington, D.C.: U.S. Dept. of Justice, National Institute of Justice : For sale by the Supt. of Docs., U.S. Govt. Print. Off.

Garland, David. 2001. *The Culture of Control: Crime and Social Order in Contemporary Society.* University of California Press.

Ghertner, Robin, and Lincoln Groves. 2018. "The Opioid Crisis and Economic Opportunity: Geographic and Economic Trends." 22.

Gibbs, Jack P. 1975. *Crime, Punishment, and Deterrence.* Elsevier.

Giddens, Anthony. 1984. *The Constitution of Society: Outline of the Theory of Structuration.* University of California Press.

Giordano, Peggy C., Stephen A. Cernkovich, and Jennifer L. Rudolph. 2002. "Gender, Crime, and Desistance: Toward a Theory of Cognitive Transformation." *American Journal of Sociology* 107(4):990–1064.

Glueck, Sheldon, and Eleanor T. Glueck. 1950. *Unraveling Juvenile Delinquency.* New York: Commonwealth Fund.

Goldstein, P. J. 1985. "The Drugs/Violence Nexus: A Tripartite Conceptual Framework." *Journal of Drug Issues* 15(4):493–506.

Goldstein, Rita Z., and Nora D. Volkow. 2002. "Drug Addiction and Its Underlying Neurobiological Basis: Neuroimaging Evidence for the Involvement of the Frontal Cortex." *American Journal of Psychiatry* 159(10):1642–52.

Goldstein, Rita Z., and Nora D. Volkow. 2011. "Dysfunction of the Prefrontal Cortex in Addiction: Neuroimaging Findings and Clinical Implications." *Nature Reviews Neuroscience* 12(11):652–69.

Gordon, Alistair M. 1973. "Patterns of Delinquency in Drug Addiction." *The British Journal of Psychiatry* 122(567):205–10.

Gottfredson, Michael R., and Travis Hirschi. 1990. *A General Theory of Crime*. Stanford University Press.

Gottschalk, Marie. 2006. *The Prison and the Gallows: The Politics of Mass Incarceration in America*. Cambridge University Press.

Gottschalk, Marie. 2016. *Caught: The Prison State and the Lockdown of American Politics*. Princeton University Press.

Graham, John, and Benjamin Bowling. 1995. *Young People and Crime*. Home Office.

Grant, Steven, Carlo Contoreggi, and Edythe D. London. 2000. "Drug Abusers Show Impaired Performance in a Laboratory Test of Decision Making." *Neuropsychologia* 38(8):1180–87.

Hammersley, Richard, Alasdair Forsyth, Valerie Morrison, and John B. Davies. 1989. "The Relationship Between Crime and Opioid Use." *British Journal of Addiction* 84(9):1029–43.

Hasin, Deborah S., Charles P. O'Brien, Marc Auriacombe, Guilherme Borges, Kathleen Bucholz, Alan Budney, Wilson M. Compton, Thomas Crowley, Walter Ling, Nancy M. Petry, Marc Schuckit, and Bridget F. Grant. 2013. "DSM-5 Criteria for Substance Use Disorders: Recommendations and Rationale." *American Journal of Psychiatry* 170(8):834–51.

Hayhurst, Karen P., Matthias Pierce, Matthew Hickman, Toby Seddon, Graham Dunn, John Keane, and Tim Millar. 2017. "Pathways through Opiate Use and Offending: A Systematic Review." *International Journal of Drug Policy* 39:1–13.

Helland, Eric, and Alexander Tabarrok. 2007. "Does Three Strikes Deter? A Nonparametric Estimation." *Journal of Human Resources* XLII(2):309–30.

Heyman, Gene M. 2009. *Addiction: A Disorder of Choice*. Harvard University Press.

Hirsch, Andrew Von. 1976. *Doing Justice: The Choice of Punishments : Report of the Committee for the Study of Incarceration*. Northeastern University Press.

Hirschi, Travis, and Michael Gottfredson. 1983. "Age and the Explanation of Crime." *American Journal of Sociology* 89(3):552–84.

Hollingsworth, Alex, Christopher J. Ruhm, and Kosali Simon. 2017. "Macroeconomic Conditions and Opioid Abuse." *Journal of Health Economics* 56:222–33.

Horney, Julie, and Ineke Haen Marshall. 1992. "Risk Perceptions Among Serious Offenders: The Role of Crime and Punishment*." *Criminology* 30(4):575–94.

Horney, Julie, D. Wayne Osgood, and Ineke Haen Marshall. 1995. "Criminal Careers in the Short-Term: Intra-Individual Variability in Crime and Its Relation to Local Life Circumstances." *American Sociological Review* 60(5):655–73.

Horwitz, Allan V., and Helene Raskin White. 1987. "Gender Role Orientations and Styles of Pathology Among Adolescents." *Journal of Health and Social Behavior* 28(2):158–70.

Hunt, Dana E., Douglas S. Lipton, and Barry Spunt. 1984. "Patterns Of Criminal Activity Among Methadone Clients And Current Narcotics Users Not in Treatment." *Journal of Drug Issues* 14:687–702.

Inciardi, James A. 1979. "Heroin Use and Street Crime." *Crime & Delinquency* 25(3):335–46.

Jalal, Hawre, Jeanine M. Buchanich, Mark S. Roberts, Lauren C. Balmert, Kun Zhang, and Donald S. Burke. 2018. "Changing Dynamics of the Drug Overdose Epidemic in the United States from 1979 through 2016." *Science* 361(6408).

Johnson, Hal, Leonard Paulozzi, Christina Porucznik, Karin Mack, and Blake Herter. 2014. "Decline in Drug Overdose Deaths After State Policy Changes — Florida, 2010–2012." *MMWR. Morbidity and Mortality Weekly Report* 63(26):569–74.

Kalivas, P. W., and J. E. Alesdatter. 1993. "Involvement of N-Methyl-D-Aspartate Receptor Stimulation in the Ventral Tegmental Area and Amygdala in Behavioral Sensitization to Cocaine." *Journal of Pharmacology and Experimental Therapeutics* 267(1):486–95.

Kay, Christopher, and Mark Monaghan. 2019. "Rethinking Recovery and Desistance Processes: Developing a Social Identity Model of Transition." *Addiction Research & Theory* 27(1):47–54.

Kaye, Sharlene, Shane Darke, and Robert Finlay-Jones. 1998. "The Onset of Heroin Use and Criminal Behaviour: Does Order Make a Difference?" *Drug and Alcohol Dependence* 53(1):79–86.

Kelly, Brian C., Mike Vuolo, and Alexandra C. Marin. 2017. "Multiple Dimensions of Peer Effects and Deviance: The Case of Prescription Drug Misuse among Young Adults." *Socius* 3:2378023117706819.

Kennedy-Hendricks, Alene, Matthew Richey, Emma E. McGinty, Elizabeth A. Stuart, Colleen L. Barry, and Daniel W. Webster. 2015. "Opioid Overdose Deaths and Florida's Crackdown on Pill Mills." *American Journal of Public Health* 106(2):291–97.

Kessler, Daniel, and Steven D. Levitt. 1999. "Using Sentence Enhancements to Distinguish Between Deterrence and Incapacitation." *The Journal of Law & Economics* 42(S1):343–64.

King, Ryan D., Michael Massoglia, and Ross Macmillan. 2007. "The Context of Marraige and Crime: Gender, the Propensity to Marry, and Offending in Early Adulthood." *Criminology* 45(1):33–65.

Kirby, Kris N., Nancy M. Petry, and Warren K. Bickel. 1999. "Heroin Addicts Have Higher Discount Rates for Delayed Rewards than Non-Drug-Using Controls." *Journal of Experimental Psychology: General* 128(1):78.

Klick, Jonathan, and Alexander Tabarrok. 2005. "Using Terror Alert Levels to Estimate the Effect of Police on Crime." *The Journal of Law and Economics* 48(1):267–79.

Kubrin, Charis E., Steven F. Messner, Glenn Deane, Kelly Mcgeever, and Thomas D. Stucky. 2010. "Proactive Policing and Robbery Rates Across U.S. Cities*." *Criminology* 48(1):57–97.

Kuhns, Joseph B., Kathleen M. Heide, and Ira Silverman. 1992. "Substance Use/Misuse among Female Prostitutes and Female Arrestees." *Substance Use and Misuse* 27(11):1283–92.

Laporte, Audrey, Adrian Rohit Dass, and Brian S. Ferguson. 2017. "Is the Rational Addiction Model Inherently Impossible to Estimate?" *Journal of Health Economics* 54:161–75.

Laub, John H., and Robert J. Sampson. 1993. "Turning Points in the Life Course: Why Change Matters to the Study of Crime*." *Criminology* 31(3):301–25.

Laub, John H., and Robert J. Sampson. 2003. *Shared Beginnings, Divergent Lives*. Harvard University Press.

Lavine, Rick. 1997. "Psychopharmacological Treatment of Aggression and Violence in the Substance Using Population." *Journal of Psychoactive Drugs* 29(4):320–29.

Lembke, Anna. 2016. *Drug Dealer, MD: How Doctors Were Duped, Patients Got Hooked, and Why It's So Hard to Stop*. JHU Press.

Lenardson, Jennifer, John Gale, and Erika Ziller. 2016. "Rural Opioid Abuse: Prevalence and User Characteristics." *Mental Health / Substance Use Disorders*.

Levitt, Steven D. 1997. "Using Electoral Cycles in Police Hiring to Estimate the Effect of Police on Crime." *American Economic Review* 87(3):270–90.

Loeber, Sabine, Theodora Duka, Helga Welzel, Helmut Nakovics, Andreas Heinz, Herta Flor, and Karl Mann. 2009. "Impairment of Cognitive Abilities and Decision Making after Chronic Use of Alcohol: The Impact of Multiple Detoxifications." *Alcohol and Alcoholism* 44(4):372–81.

MacDonald, John M. 2002. "The Effectiveness of Community Policing in Reducing Urban Violence." *Crime & Delinquency* 48(4):592–618.

MacKillop, James, Michael T. Amlung, Lauren R. Few, Lara A. Ray, Lawrence H. Sweet, and Marcus R. Munafò. 2011. "Delayed Reward Discounting and Addictive Behavior: A Meta-Analysis." *Psychopharmacology* 216(3):305–21.

Marel, Christina, Katherine L. Mills, Shane Darke, Joanne Ross, Tim Slade, Lucy Burns, and Maree Teesson. 2013. "Static and Dynamic Predictors of Criminal Involvement among People with Heroin Dependence: Findings from a 3-Year Longitudinal Study." *Drug and Alcohol Dependence* 133(2):600–606.

Maruna, Shadd. 2001. *Making Good: How Ex-Convicts Reform and Rebuild Their Lives.* American Psychological Association.

Marvell, Thomas B., and Carlisle E. Moody. 1996. "Specification Problems, Police Levels, and Crime Rates*." *Criminology* 34(4):609–46.

Massoglia, Michael, and Christopher Uggen. 2010. "Settling Down and Aging Out: Toward an Interactionist Theory of Desistance and the Transition to Adulthood." *American Journal of Sociology* 116(2):543–82.

Matsueda, Ross L., Derek A. Kreager, and David Huizinga. 2006. "Deterring Delinquents: A Rational Choice Model of Theft and Violence." *American Sociological Review* 71(1):95–122.

Matza, David. 1964. *Delinquency and Drift*. Transaction Publishers.

McBride, Duane C., and Clyde B. McCoy. 1981. "Crime and Drug-Using Behavior." *Criminology* 19(2):281–302.

McIntosh, James, and Neil McKeageny. 2002. *Beating the Dragon: The Recovery from Dependent Drug Use*. Routledge.

Meier, Robert F., and Weldon T. Johnson. 1977. "Deterrence as Social Control: The Legal and Extralegal Production of Conformity." *American Sociological Review* 42(2):292–304.

Melberg, Hans O., and Ole J. Rogeberg. 2008. "Rational Addiction Theory: A Survey of Opinions." *Journal of Drug Policy Analysis* 3(1).

Merton, Robert K. 1938. "Social Structure and Anomie." *American Sociological Review* 3(5):672–82.

Messner, Steven F., Sandro Galea, Kenneth J. Tardiff, Melissa Tracy, Angela Bucciarelli, Tinka Markham Piper, Victoria Frye, and David Vlahov. 2007. "Policing, Drugs, and the Homicide Decline in New York City in the 1990s." *Criminology* 45(2):385–414.

Messner, Steven F., and Richard Rosenfeld. 1994. *Crime and the American Dream*. Cengage Learning.

Mitchell, Ojmarrh, Joshua C. Cochran, Daniel P. Mears, and William D. Bales. 2017. "The Effectiveness of Prison for Reducing Drug Offender Recidivism: A Regression Discontinuity Analysis." *Journal of Experimental Criminology* 13(1):1–27.

Monnat, Shannon M. 2018. "The Contributions of Socioeconomic and Opioid Supply Factors to U.S. Drug Mortality Rates: Urban-Rural and within-Rural Differences." *Journal of Rural Studies*.

Monnat, Shannon M., and Khary K. Rigg. 2016. "Examining Rural/Urban Differences in Prescription Opioid Misuse Among US Adolescents." *The Journal of Rural Health* 32(2):204–18.

Murakawa, Naomi, and Katherine Beckett. 2010. "The Penology of Racial Innocence: The Erasure of Racism in the Study and Practice of Punishment." *Law & Society Review* 44(3–4):695–730.

Myers, Catherine E., Jony Sheynin, Tarryn Balsdon, Andre Luzardo, Kevin D. Beck, Lee Hogarth, Paul Haber, and Ahmed A. Moustafa. 2016. "Probabilistic Reward- and Punishment-Based Learning in Opioid Addiction: Experimental and Computational Data." *Behavioural Brain Research* 296:240–48.

Nagin, Daniel S. 1998. "Criminal Deterrence Research at the Outset of the Twenty-First Century." *Crime and Justice* 23:1–42.

Nagin, Daniel S. 2013. "Deterrence: A Review of the Evidence by a Criminologist for Economists." *Annual Review of Economics* 5(1):83–105.

Nagin, Daniel S., and G. Matthew Snodgrass. 2013. "The Effect of Incarceration on Re-Offending: Evidence from a Natural Experiment in Pennsylvania." *Journal of Quantitative Criminology* 29(4):601–42.

Nurco, David N., John W. Shaffer, John C. Ball, and Timothy W. Kinlock. 1984. "Trends in the Commission of Crime among Narcotic Addicts over Successive Periods of Addiction and Nonaddiction (Informa Healthcare)." *The American Journal of Drug and Alcohol Abuse* 10(4):481–89.

O'Brien, Charles P. 2003. "Research Advances in the Understanding and Treatment of Addiction." *The American Journal on Addictions* 12(s2):S36–47.

Olekalns, Nilss, and Peter Bardsley. 1996. "Rational Addiction to Caffeine: An Analysis of Coffee Consumption." *Journal of Political Economy* 104(5):1100–1104.

Orphanides, Athanasios, and David Zervos. 1995. "Rational Addiction with Learning and Regret." *Journal of Political Economy* 103(4):739.

Orphanides, Athanasios, and David Zervos. 1998. "Myopia and Addictive Behaviour." *The Economic Journal* 108(446):75–91.

Palombi, Laura C., Catherine A. St Hill, Martin S. Lipsky, Michael T. Swanoski, and M. Nawal Lutfiyya. 2018. "A Scoping Review of Opioid Misuse in the Rural United States." *Annals of Epidemiology* 28(9):641–52.

Paternoster, R., and S. Bushway. 2009. "Desistance and the 'Feared Self': Toward an Identity Theory of Criminal Desistance." *Journal of Criminal Law and Criminology* 99(4):1103–56.

Paulozzi, Leonard J. 2006. "Opioid Analgesic Involvement in Drug Abuse Deaths in American Metropolitan Areas." *American Journal of Public Health* 96(10):1755–57.

Paulozzi, Leonard J., Edwin M. Kilbourne, and Hema A. Desai. 2011. "Prescription Drug Monitoring Programs and Death Rates from Drug Overdose." *Pain Medicine* 12(5):747–54.

Perry, Amanda E., Matthew Neilson, Marrissa Martyn-St James, Julie M. Glanville, Rebecca Woodhouse, Christine Godfrey, and Catherine Hewitt. 2015. "Interventions for Drug-using Offenders with Co-occurring Mental Illness." *Cochrane Database of Systematic Reviews* (6).

Petersilia, Joan. 2003. *When Prisoners Come Home: Parole and Prisoner Reentry*. Oxford University Press.

PEW Charitable Trusts. 2018. *More Imprisonment Does Not Reduce State Drug Problems.*

Pickard, Hanna. 2018. "The Puzzle of Addiction." Pp. 9–22 in *The Routledge Handbook of Philosophy and Science of Addiction*, edited by H. Pickard and S. H. Ahmed. 1 [edition]. | New York : Routledge, 2018. | Series: Routledge handbooks in philosophy: Routledge.

Piliavin, Irving, Rosemary Gartner, Craig Thornton, and Ross L. Matsueda. 1986. "Crime, Deterrence, and Rational Choice." *American Sociological Review* 51(1):101–19.

Pirastu, R., R. Fais, M. Messina, V. Bini, S. Spiga, D. Falconieri, and M. Diana. 2006. "Impaired Decision-Making in Opiate-Dependent Subjects: Effect of Pharmacological Therapies." *Drug and Alcohol Dependence* 83(2):163–68.

Pogarsky, Greg. 2002. "Identifying 'Deterrable' Offenders: Implications for Research on Deterrence." *Justice Quarterly* 19(3):431–52.

Pogarsky, Greg, and Alex R. Piquero. 2003. "Can Punishment Encourage Offending? Investigating The 'Resetting' Effect." *Journal of Research in Crime and Delinquency* 40(1):95–120.

Qiu, Ying-wei, Gui-hua Jiang, Huan-huan Su, Xiao-fei Lv, Jun-zhang Tian, Li-ming Li, and Fu-zhen Zhuo. 2013. "The Impulsivity Behavior Is Correlated with Prefrontal Cortex Gray Matter Volume Reduction in Heroin-Dependent Individuals." *Neuroscience Letters* 538:43–48.

Redish, A. David, Steve Jensen, and Adam Johnson. 2008. "A Unified Framework for Addiction: Vulnerabilities in the Decision Process." *Behavioral and Brain Sciences* 31(4):415–37.

Remillard, Daniel, Alan David Kaye, and Heath McAnally. 2019. "Oxycodone's Unparalleled Addictive Potential: Is It Time for a Moratorium?" *Current Pain and Headache Reports* 23(2):15.

Rigg, Khary K., Samantha J. March, and James A. Inciardi. 2010. "Prescription Drug Abuse & Diversion: Role of the Pain Clinic." *Journal of Drug Issues* 40(3):681–701.

Rigg, Khary K., Shannon M. Monnat, and Melody N. Chavez. 2018. "Opioid-Related Mortality in Rural America: Geographic Heterogeneity and Intervention Strategies." *International Journal of Drug Policy* 57:119–29.

Rogeberg, Ole. 2020. "The Theory of Rational Addiction." *Addiction* 115(1):184–87.

Rogeberg, Ole, and Hans Olav Melberg. 2011. "Acceptance of Unsupported Claims about Reality: A Blind Spot in Economics." *Journal of Economic Methodology* 18(01):29–52.

Rowlands, David, Donna Youngs, and David Canter. 2020. "Agency and Communion: Modeling Identity-Transformation in Recovery from Substance Misuse." *Journal of Substance Use* 25(2):163–72.

Rubin, Herbert J., and Irene S. Rubin. 2012. *Qualitative Interviewing: The Art of Hearing Data.* SAGE Publications.

Rudd, R. A., N. Aleshire, J. E. Zibbell, and R. Matthew Gladden. 2016. "Increases in Drug and Opioid Overdose Deaths—United States, 2000–2014." *American Journal of Transplantation* 16(4):1323–27.

Rutkow, Lainie, Hsien-Yen Chang, Matthew Daubresse, Daniel W. Webster, Elizabeth A. Stuart, and G. Caleb Alexander. 2015. "Effect of Florida's Prescription Drug Monitoring Program and Pill Mill Laws on Opioid Prescribing and Use." *JAMA Internal Medicine* 175(10):1642–49.

Saddoris, Michael P., Fabio Cacciapaglia, R. Mark Wightman, and Regina M. Carelli. 2015. "Differential Dopamine Release Dynamics in the Nucleus Accumbens Core and Shell Reveal Complementary Signals for Error Prediction and Incentive Motivation." *Journal of Neuroscience* 35(33):11572–82.

Sampson, Robert J., and Jacqueline Cohen. 1988. "Deterrent Effects of the Police on Crime: A Replication and Theoretical Extension." *Law & Society Review* 22(1):163–89.

Sampson, Robert J., and John H. Laub. 1990. "Crime and Deviance over the Life Course: The Salience of Adult Social Bonds." *American Sociological Review* 55(5):609–27.

Sampson, Robert J., and John H. Laub. 1993. *Crime in the Making: Pathways and Turning Points Through Life*. Harvard University Press.

Satel, Sally, and Scott O. Lilienfeld. 2013. *Brainwashed: The Seductive Appeal of Mindless Neuroscience*. Basic Books.

Senay, Edward C. 1999. "Neurobiology of Opiates and Opioids." Pp. 271–79 in *Textbook of substance abuse treatment*, edited by M. Galanter and H. Kleber. Washington, D.C.: American Psychiatric Press.

Shepherd, Joanna M. 2002. "Fear of the First Strike: The Full Deterrent Effect of California's Two- and Three-Strikes Legislation." *The Journal of Legal Studies* 31(1):159–201.

Sherman, Lawrence W. 1990. "Police Crackdowns: Initial and Residual Deterrence." *Crime and Justice* 12:1–48.

Sherman, Lawrence W., Douglas A. Smith, Janell D. Schmidt, and Dennis P. Rogan. 1992. "Crime, Punishment, and Stake in Conformity: Legal and Informal Control of Domestic Violence." *American Sociological Review* 57(5):680–90.

Sisto, Andrea, and Roberto Zanola. 2010. "Cinema Attendance in Europe." *Applied Economics Letters* 17(5):515–517.

Skardhamar, TorbjøRn, and Jukka Savolainen. 2014. "Changes in Criminal Offending Around the Time of Job Reentry: A Study of Employment and Desistance: Timing of Employment and Desistance." *Criminology* 52(2):263–91.

Smith, David E. 2017. "Medicalizing the Opioid Epidemic in the U.S. in the Era of Health Care Reform." *Journal of Psychoactive Drugs* 49(2):95–101.

Smyth, BP, J. Barry, E. Keenan, and K. Ducray. 2010. "Lapse and Relapse Following Inpatient Treatment of Opiate Dependence." *The Irish Medical Journal* 103(6):176–79.

Spenner, Erin LeAnne, Aju J. Fenn, and John R. Crooker. 2010. "The Demand For NFL Attendance: A Rational Addiction Model." *Journal of Business & Economics Research (JBER)* 8(12).

Stafford, Mark C., and Mark Warr. 1993. "- A Reconceptualization of General and Specific Deterrence." *Journal of Research in Crime and Delinquency* 30(2):123–35.

Stewart, Jennifer L., Mamona Butt, April C. May, Susan F. Tapert, and Martin P. Paulus. 2017. "Insular and Cingulate Attenuation during Decision Making Is Associated with Future Transition to Stimulant Use Disorder." *Addiction* 112(9):1567–77.

Stewart, Jennifer L., Taru M. Flagan, April C. May, Martina Reske, Alan N. Simmons, and Martin P. Paulus. 2013. "Young Adults at Risk for Stimulant Dependence Show Reward Dysfunction During Reinforcement-Based Decision Making." *Biological Psychiatry* 73(3):235–41.

Stolzenberg, Lisa, and Stewart J. D'Alessio. 1997. "'Three Strikes and You're Out': The Impact of California's New Mandatory Sentencing Law on Serious Crime Rates." *Crime & Delinquency* 43(4):457–69.

The Sentencing Project. 2018. *Report to the United Nations on Racial Disparities in the U.S. Criminal Justice System*. Washington D.C.

Tobler, Philippe N., Katrin H. Preller, Daniel K. Campbell-Meiklejohn, Matthias Kirschner, Rainer Kraehenmann, Philipp Stämpfli, Marcus Herdener, Erich Seifritz, and Boris B. Quednow. 2016. "Shared Neural Basis of Social and Non-Social Reward Deficits in Chronic Cocaine Users." *Social Cognitive and Affective Neuroscience* 11(6):1017–25.

Tonry, Michael. 2008. "Learning from the Limitations of Deterrence Research." *Crime and Justice* 37(1):279–311.

Trifilieff, P., B. Feng, E. Urizar, V. Winiger, R. D. Ward, K. M. Taylor, D. Martinez, H. Moore, P. D. Balsam, E. H. Simpson, and J. A. Javitch. 2013. "Increasing Dopamine D2 Receptor Expression in the Adult Nucleus Accumbens Enhances Motivation." *Molecular Psychiatry* 18(9):1025–33.

Turpeinen, Pirkko. 2001. "Outcome of Drug Abuse in a 20-Year Follow-up Study of Drug-Experimenting Schoolchildren in Finland." *Nordic Journal of Psychiatry* 55(4):263–70.

Uggen, Christopher. 2000. "Work as a Turning Point in the Life Course of Criminals: A Duration Model of Age, Employment, and Recidivism." *American Sociological Review* 65(4):529–46.

Verdejo-García, Antonio, Miguel A. Alcázar-Córcoles, and Natalia Albein-Urios. 2019. "Neuropsychological Interventions for Decision-Making in Addiction: A Systematic Review." *Neuropsychology Review* 29(1):79–92.

Verdejo-Garcia, Antonio, Amy Benbrook, Frank Funderburk, Paula David, Jean-Lud Cadet, and Karen I. Bolla. 2007. "The Differential Relationship between Cocaine Use and Marijuana Use on Decision-Making Performance over Repeat Testing with the Iowa Gambling Task." *Drug and Alcohol Dependence* 90(1):2–11.

Volkow, Nora, Helene Benveniste, and A. Thomas McLellan. 2018. "Use and Misuse of Opioids in Chronic Pain." *Annual Review of Medicine* 69(1):451–65.

Volkow, Nora D., George F. Koob, and A. Thomas McLellan. 2016. "Neurobiologic Advances from the Brain Disease Model of Addiction." *New England Journal of Medicine* 374(4):363–71.

Vonmoos, Matthias, Lea M. Hulka, Katrin H. Preller, Daniela Jenni, Markus R. Baumgartner, Rudolf Stohler, Karen I. Bolla, and Boris B. Quednow. 2013. "Cognitive Dysfunctions in Recreational and Dependent Cocaine Users: Role of Attention-Deficit Hyperactivity Disorder, Craving and Early Age at Onset." *The British Journal of Psychiatry* 203(1):35–43.

Waldo, Gordon P., and Theodore G. Chiricos. 1972. "Perceived Penal Sanction and Self-Reported Criminality: A Neglected Approach to Deterrence Research." *Social Problems* 19(4):522–40.

Wang, Shaocheng. 2019. "Historical Review: Opiate Addiction and Opioid Receptors." *Cell Transplantation* 28(3):233–38.

Wang, Xuyi, Baojuan Li, Xuhui Zhou, Yanhui Liao, Jinsong Tang, Tieqiao Liu, Dewen Hu, and Wei Hao. 2012. "Changes in Brain Gray Matter in Abstinent Heroin Addicts." *Drug and Alcohol Dependence* 126(3):304–8.

Webster, Cheryl Marie, Anthony N. Doob, and Franklin E. Zimring. 2006. "Proposition 8 and Crime Rates in California: The Case of the Disappearing Deterrent." *Criminology & Public Policy* 5(3):417–48.

Weisberg, Daniel F., William C. Becker, David A. Fiellin, and Cathy Stannard. 2014. "Prescription Opioid Misuse in the United States and the United Kingdom: Cautionary Lessons." *International Journal of Drug Policy* 25(6):1124–30.

Weissman, James C., Paul L. Katsampes, and Thomas A. Giacinti. 1974. "Opiate Use and Criminality among a Jail Population." *Addictive Diseases: An International Journal* 1(3):269–81.

Williams, Kirk R., and Richard Hawkins. 1986. "Perceptual Research on General Deterrence: A Critical Review." *Law & Society Review* 20(4):545–72.

Wilson, James Q., and Barbara Boland. 1978. "The Effect of the Police on Crime." *Law & Society Review* 12(3):367–90.

Wilson, James Q., and George L. Kelling. 1982. "Broken Windows." *Atlantic Monthly*, 29–38.

Wise, Roy A. 2002. "Brain Reward Circuitry: Insights from Unsensed Incentives." *Neuron* 36(2):229–40.

Zijlstra, Fleur, Jan Booij, Wim van den Brink, and Ingmar H. A. Franken. 2008. "Striatal Dopamine D2 Receptor Binding and Dopamine Release during Cue-Elicited Craving in Recently Abstinent Opiate-Dependent Males." *European Neuropsychopharmacology* 18(4):262–70.

Appendix A: Interview Guide

Context
1. Can you tell me about where you're from? How would you describe it?
   - Know people? Did they know you?
   - Economic stability?
     - o Able to find work if you wanted it?
   - Did people move in and out a lot?
   - Were people losing their homes or moving around a lot?
   - Was there much crime there?

2. Can you tell me about opioid use in your community?
   - Do you think that it was it common? Uncommon?

   - Was there a time where you started to notice that opioids were becoming more of a thing where you lived?

   - How did people you know talk about opioids?
     - o Did people think it was a problem?

   - How long had you lived there?
     - o Had it changed over time (e.g., business closing, new apartment buildings, etc.)?
     - o <u>(If Bad)</u>: Do you think things can turn around?

3. Do you think that where you lived affected your use of drugs?
   - Starting, stopping, etc.
   - Might have been different if elsewhere?

4. What kinds of treatment options did you have where you lived?
   - Do you think people would have judged you if you wanted to get treatment?

Life Circumstances, the Development of Use, and Turning Points
5. Can you describe the time when you first used opioids?
   - How were you introduced you to them?
   - How did you (or they) get them?

   - What was going on in your life around this time?
     - o Were there things that you were happy about?
       - ▪ Sad or upset?

223

o Were there any stressful events going on around this time?
- Were any of those things related to friends or family, rather than yourself?
- How do you think these things affected you?
- How did you handle or cope with these problems?

7. When was the second time that you used?
- Can you tell me more about how much you were using in the days and weeks after that?
- Did you start to feel like you had an addiction?
  o When? What made you feel that way?
- Did you ever have physical symptoms/sickness like withdrawals?
  o When? How did those make you feel?

8. In your mind, were there different stages of your use? (e.g., severity of drugs, switching from smoking to injecting)
- What was behind changes in how much you used or how you used?
  o Frequency of use?
  o Why do you think your use escalated?
  o Were you using other drugs at the same time?
- Rx opioids?

- (If Rx used) Did you experience any kind of increased regulation of the prescriptions, like a drug management program?
  o Were you aware of any increased regulations while you were on the medication?
  o Did it get easier or harder for you to get your drugs over time? How so?

9. What did your drug use mean for you?
- Was it about partying? Feeling good?
  o What about for other people you knew?
- Did you ever talk about it with anyone else?

10. Did your drug use ever interfere with work or your ability to hold a job/find a job?
- How was your financial situation before you started using?
  o How about your family's?
- How were you supporting yourself during your addiction?
  o During recovery?
- How would you compare your average day during periods of use to before you started using?

11. Did you ever have any overdoses?
- How did your thinking about your drug use change at all?
- Did you feel any different?

12. Were you ever around overdoses?
- Was it people that you knew well?
  o Friends or family?

- What would you do if that happened? Did you call anyone?
  o How long did it take for them to get there?

- Did these experiences affect your drug use?

- Any naloxone-related experiences? Personal or otherwise?

13. How did you progress into not using anymore?
- What was the first step?

- Did you have setbacks or relapses on the way?
  o Did you try to stop or cut back more than once?
  o Have you had several periods of sobriety?

- Was there a specific moment that you remember when you decided you wanted to quit?

- How much of this decision was your choice?

14. Did anyone that you hung out with or spent time with also use drugs?
- Did people that you spent time with or hang out with change over the course of your drug use?
  o Since you began recovery?

- Has your network of friends or family changed since you've been in recovery?
  o Do you think it will change in the future?

15. Were there people that you tried to hide your drug use from?
- Why or why not?

Strain

16. Were you happy with how successful you were in life around the time you started using drugs?

- Can you give me an idea of what success look like to you?
  - o Are there specific things or goals that you needed to think of yourself as a success?

- How about in comparison to friends, family? Within your community?
  - o Did you ever make those comparisons?
  - o Were there ever things that made you feel like others higher status than you?

- How did your situation make you feel?
  - o Content? Discouraged? Angry?

- Did you feel pressure to be successful?

- Did you ever wish that you had more?

- Have you or your family had any financial obstacles?

- Before you started using, how would you compare where you were to where you wanted to be?
  - o Were they the same? Different?
  - o How about after you started using?

18. Do you feel like you had control over where you went in life? Do you feel like your path was sort of pre-determined?
- How about now?

19. Did you feel like you had the opportunity to achieve your goals or get what you wanted in life?
- NO: How did that make you feel? Did it change the things that you did?
- YES: What sorts of opportunities do you think you had?

Perception of Legal Consequences and the Influence of Criminal Justice Contact
20. When you were in your addiction, were you ever worried about being arrested?
- Yes
  - o How did you think about the possibility that you'd end up getting arrested?
    - ▪ Was it something you thought about much?
      - • Did it matter to you or have any impact on the things that you did?

- Were there things that, in your mind, you could do to make it less likely that you'd get arrested?
  - Change what drugs you used?
  - Change where you got them?
- How did you think about the prospect of serving time?
  - Was that ever something that changed your behavior?

- Was the thought of being arrested something that worried you?
  - What worried you?
  - Things you were afraid of losing?
  - Legal troubles of people you know? Friends/family?
  - Did worries alter your drug use?

- Were you aware of any police efforts that were targeting opioids?
  - How about any changes to sentencing or anything like that?

21. (If ever arrested) How has/have your arrest(s) influenced your drug use?
- Has it reduced or stopped it?
  - Did it take multiple arrests to change things for you?
  - No reductions?
- What was going on around the time you were first arrested?
- As you were arrested more, did it change your thinking about the risks of use?

Recovery and Policy Implications

26. Can you tell me about your recovery process? How has it been for you?
- Different periods of sobriety and relapses?
  - detox or rehab programs?
    - How many?

- What have been some of the most important influences in your recovery?

- What kinds of other resources, support activities, or groups have you utilized?
  - Currently?
  - What aspects of programs have been helpful for you? Not as helpful?

- What have been some of the challenges or obstacles during your recovery?

- Have you dealt with cravings?
  - How do you handle those situations when they come up?

27. Do you think that drug addiction is an illness?

28. What do you think that policymakers and the police could do to help people struggling with addiction? What would you tell them?
- What do you think they should know that they might not already know?